INJECTION TECHNIQUES
in Orthopaedic
and Sports Medicine

A practical manual for doctors
and physiotherapists

D1244257

Dedication

In memory of Peter – my generous partner and best friend.

For Elsevier:

Senior Commissioning Editor: Sarena Wolfaard
Development Editor: Claire Wilson
Project Manager: Caroline Horton, Morven Dean
Design: George Ajayi
Illustration Manager: Bruce Hogarth
Illustrator: Amanda Williams

INJECTION TECHNIQUES

in Orthopaedic and Sports Medicine

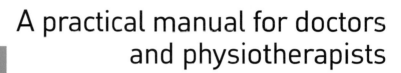

A practical manual for doctors and physiotherapists

THIRD EDITION

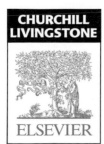

Stephanie Saunders FCSP FSOM

Private Practitioner; Course Director, Orthopaedic Medicine Seminars and the Association of Chartered Physiotherapists in Orthopaedic Medicine;
Fellow of Chartered Society of Physiotherapists, London, UK

Steve Longworth MB ChB MSc FRCGP DM-SMED DPCR FSOM

Principal in General Practice, East Leicester Medical Practice,
Uppingham Road Health Centre, Leicester, UK

Foreword by
Peter Maddison MD FRCP

Consultant Rheumatologist, North West Wales and Professor of Joint and Muscle Disorders, School of Sport, Health and Exercise Science, University of Wales, Bangor, UK

CHURCHILL LIVINGSTONE

ELSEVIER

EDINBURGH LONDON NEW YORK OXFORD PHILADELPHIA
ST LOUIS SYDNEY TORONTO 2006

ELSEVIER | CHURCHILL LIVINGSTONE

An imprint of Elsevier Limited

First edition 1997
Second edition 2002
Third edition 2006

ISBN-10 0443 074984
ISBN-13 978 0443 07498 1

British Library Cataloguing in Publication Data
A catalogue record for this book is available from the British Library

Library of Congress Cataloging in Publication Data
A catalog record for this book is available from the Library of Congress

Notice
Knowledge and best practice in this field are constantly changing. As new research and experience broaden our knowledge, changes in practice, treatment and drug therapy may become necessary or appropriate. Readers are advised to check the most current information provided (i) on procedures featured or (ii) by the manufacturer of each product to be administered, to verify the recommended dose or formula, the method and duration of administration, and contraindications. It is the responsibility of the practitioner, relying on their own experience and knowledge of the patient, to make diagnoses, to determine dosages and the best treatment for each individual patient, and to take all appropriate safety precautions. To the fullest extent of the law, neither the Publisher nor the Authors assume any liability for any injury and/or damage to persons or property arising out of or related to any use of the material contained in this book.

The Publisher

ELSEVIER your source for books, journals and multimedia in the health sciences

www.elsevierhealth.com

The publisher's policy is to use paper manufactured from sustainable forests

Printed in China by CTPS

Contents

The CD-ROM accompanying this text includes video sequences of all the techniques indicated in the text by the icon. To look at the video for a given technique, click on the relevant icon in the contents list on the CD-ROM. The CD-ROM is designed to be used in conjunction with the text and not as a stand-alone product.

Foreword

The ability to aspirate joints and perform accurate articular and periarticular injections is an essential skill in managing people with musculoskeletal disorders. This manual is an outstanding reference not only for practitioners who are embarking on developing these skills but also for those of us who need a reminder about the less commonly performed injection techniques.

Stephanie Saunders, now collaborating with Dr Steve Longworth, has improved on her original book with every new edition. This third edition is the best yet and is an exceptionally informative book covering a very wide range of specific techniques. It is written in a scholarly way and provides a good background of clinical evidence. For those who like obscure references there are plenty here. However, it remains a highly practical manual with lots of good illustrations and helpful flow charts and summary tables. This edition also comes with a CD-ROM, which is a very useful visual aid to performing the techniques.

This book will appeal to the broad range of practitioners who are developing joint and soft tissue injection techniques. It is essential reading for doctors, physiotherapists, nurses and other health professionals involved in managing musculoskeletal disorders and sports injuries, whether in the context of primary or secondary care.

Peter Maddison, January 2006

Preface

This is the third edition of *Injection Techniques in Orthopaedic and Sports Medicine*. When I first started using injection therapy for the treatment of musculoskeletal pain, there was no simple text on approaches, doses and techniques for this therapeutic skill. Most of my knowledge of the subject was gained from Dr James Cyriax, with whom I worked and taught for many years, and to whom I shall always be indebted. The rest was worked out by trial and error using long-suffering patients and colleagues as aids, and by scouring vast medical textbooks looking for consistent information on the subject.

When, in 1995, I started teaching courses on injection therapy specifically to chartered physiotherapists, I was persuaded that there was a place for a simple, easy-to-follow guide for both medical practitioners and physiotherapists, and so the forerunner to this book was born. It has now grown from a small manual to a deeply referenced textbook on the subject, but still with the object of keeping the information simple.

I have been joined in this edition by Dr Steve Longworth, co-tutor on the courses and a most enthusiastic and diligent co-author. I am extremely indebted to his tenacity in digging up the most obscure of references, and spending many hours fiddling with bits of text – usually when I thought the final, final draft had been finished.

The evidence has been updated and several new techniques added, and the CD-ROM which accompanies the text provides a useful visual aid to assist the clinician in performing the techniques.

We have been most encouraged by the enthusiastic response from our students and colleagues, and it is they who have put forward ideas and constructive criticism for this new edition. Patients, and the results they have reported, have also contributed to the final result. Lynne Gardner, my patient secretary; Claire Wilson, equally patient editor; Carrie Horton, uncomplaining project manager; Elizabeth Kerridge Weeks, excellent proof reader; Cameron Mather and his expert team who made filming for the CD-ROM such an entertaining experience; and Andrew Maclain, our long-suffering model, made this edition possible. To all of them we extend our thanks.

We hope you enjoy reading this book, that the skills contained herein will provide your patients with the pain relief they are seeking, and that their gratitude will give you as much satisfaction and pleasure as it does us.

Stephanie Saunders
London, May 2006

The evidence base for injection therapy

Injection therapy is the treatment of musculoskeletal disorders by the localized injection of a drug, usually a corticosteroid and a local anaesthetic. It has been in use for more than 50 years and there is a wealth of anecdotal evidence of its efficacy. Despite this, there are few definitive studies of its application in joint and soft tissue lesions[1-3,199] and few studies comparing injection therapy with other treatments[4,6-8,17,105,244-246]. This is surprising because injection therapy is the most common therapeutic intervention in rheumatological practice[265]. Consequently there are few facts and a mass of opinions – many of them dogmatic and contradictory – about almost every aspect of injection therapy[9,150].

Interpretation of injection therapy studies is compounded by a disconcerting lack of expert agreement about definitions, diagnosis and outcome measures in musculoskeletal medicine[10,11,17,18,148,155,247,253,267]. Authoritative reviews tend to be conservative in their estimates of the presence and size of treatment effects in injection therapy[231,248-251,266].

Nonetheless, injection therapy is recommended for knee and shoulder problems in national and international guidelines[173,174,254], and is used extensively for other musculoskeletal conditions[32,258]. Given its relative safety[64], ease of application in trained hands, and cost-effectiveness[105], plus the frequent lack of convincing systematic evidence for the effectiveness of alternatives[231,248-251], injection therapy is a very useful treatment modality. This is supported by the collective experience of the majority of clinicians in primary care and the locomotor specialties[255].

As with other modalities, the challenge for all clinicians delivering injection therapy is to implement evidence-based practice by applying the best research-based treatments, tempered by clinical experience and patients' values[149]. Where good research evidence is lacking, clinicians should become involved in research that will provide that evidence.

Problems with injection therapy arise when:

- an *inappropriate drug* is chosen
- too *large* a dose or volume is given
- the drug is put into the *wrong tissue*
- *poor technique* allows spread of drugs to adjacent tissue
- injections are given too *frequently*
- insufficient attention is directed to the *cause* of the *lesion*
- no regard is given to *aftercare* and *rehabilitation*

The art of good injection therapy is to select the appropriate patient, and to place the minimal effective amount of an appropriate drug into the exact site of the affected tissue. This means that the clinician using injection therapy must possess a high level of diagnostic and technical skill.

CLINICIANS WHO DELIVER INJECTION THERAPY

Doctors in orthopaedics, rheumatology, pain management, musculoskeletal and sports medicine are the main medical specialists who deliver injection therapy. Just over a half of all general practitioners (GPs) also give these injections, but most of the injections in the community are performed by just 5% of GPs[273]. The main perceived barriers to performing joint and soft tissue injections by doctors in the community are inadequate training, the inability to maintain injection skills and discomfort with the performance of the technique[273,274]. Training improves GPs' injection activity and their level of confidence[275].

Since 1995, chartered physiotherapists in the United Kingdom have been offered training in the use of the injection therapy techniques described in this book. Injection therapy guidelines for physiotherapists are available[21]. Injection therapy administered by a physiotherapist has been shown to be part of a very effective way of managing orthopaedic[22] and rheumatology[23] outpatients and patients in the community with musculoskeletal problems[24]. Extended Scope Practitioners in physiotherapy have been shown to be as effective as orthopaedic surgeons and to generate lower initial direct hospital costs[25]. Nurses have also been trained in injection therapy[276,314]. Non-medical clinicians may deliver injection therapy under a Patient Group Direction (PGD).

CURRENT CONTROVERSIES IN INJECTION THERAPY

Almost every aspect of injection therapy is non-standardized. Notwithstanding controversies about diagnosis, there is no universal agreement about the following questions:

● What are we treating i.e. what is the pathological or biochemical abnormality responsible for the pain in tendinopathy?
● Are we always treating inflammation, or is the steroid, and possibly the local anaesthetic, doing something else, e.g. modifying the action of nociceptors?
● Are there subgroups of potential injection therapy responders within broad diagnostic categories such as 'shoulder pain' and 'mechanical back pain' and if so how can we identify them?
● Which steroid, local anaesthetic, dosages, volumes, injection techniques, aseptic techniques, venues (office or operating theatre), aftercare (rest or not), co-interventions and rehabilitation advice should we be advocating?
● Timing of injection therapy; when in the course of any disorder is the optimal time to inject, should injections be repeated and if so at what intervals and how often?
● Who should we follow up, at what intervals and for how long?
● How useful is the confirmation of placement of injection by imaging e.g. ultrasound scanning? (See Accuracy of injection)
● How much of the benefit of injection therapy is due to the placebo effect, the effect of needling (acupuncture) or the effect of simply injecting a

volume of fluid as opposed to any specific pharmacological effect of the drugs used?

● Which clinicians, other than doctors, should be trained in injection therapy?
● How much mythology and misinformation is there about injection therapy and how can we correct it?
● Is injected saline an analgesic[230,294]? Such an effect of saline injection into soft tissues and joints may have implications for the interpretation of previously published placebo controlled studies of intra-articular analgesia in which saline was used as an (assumed) inactive control treatment
● Can intramuscular steroid injection assist in the healing of muscle injuries? Clinical experience and laboratory experiments on non-human animal models point in opposite directions; the clinicians say 'yes', the scientists say 'no'[295,296]

For more detailed discussion of some of the controversies surrounding injection therapy see:

Speed CA. Corticosteroid injections in tendon lesions. *British Medical Journal* 2001;323:382–386.
Steve Longworth's Rapid Response on bmj.com.

Only high-quality research will answer these questions. Undoubtedly it will raise many more.

SECTION 1

GUIDELINES AND PROCEDURES

THE DRUGS

CORTICOSTEROIDS

The commonly used injectable corticosteroids are synthetic analogues of the adrenal glucocorticoid hormone cortisol (hydrocortisone), which is secreted by the innermost layer (zona reticularis) of the adrenal cortex. Cortisol has many important actions, including effects on protein and glucose metabolism, but it also has anti-inflammatory activity, which is mediated by effects on polymorph and macrophage migration and suppression of the immunological response of lymphocytes[26,27,197].

When they were first administered systemically in the 1940s steroid drugs were hailed as the new 'universal panacea', but it soon became apparent that major side-effects greatly limited their systemic use[28]. In 1951, Hollander, in the USA, reported the first use of local hydrocortisone injections for arthritic joints[29]. Virtually insoluble steroid suspensions are used because intra-articular soluble steroids will rapidly clear into the systemic circulation. The suspensions work by minute quantities of the active drug dissolving off the surface of the crystals when in contact with the inflamed tissue[28]. In joints, the steroid is taken up by the synovial cells before being gradually absorbed into the blood and cleared[1,31,261,262].

Corticosteroids exert their many effects on the cells involved in the immune and inflammatory responses primarily by modulating the transcription of a large number of genes. They act directly on nuclear steroid receptors to control the rate of synthesis of mRNA[32]. However, they also influence the mechanisms by which proteins are synthesized, and thereby affect the production of a wide range of proinflammatory mediators including cytokines[33] and other important enzymes.

RATIONALE FOR USING CORTICO-STEROIDS

We know surprisingly little about the precise pharmacological effects of corticosteroids when they are injected directly into joints and soft tissues[34,206]. Local steroid injections are thought to work by:

- *Suppressing inflammation* in inflammatory systemic diseases such as rheumatoid or psoriatic arthritis, gout, etc[28,31,34–36,194,218]

- *Suppressing inflammatory flares* in degenerative joint disease[31,32,37–40]. The classic distinction between osteoarthrosis and osteoarthritis is not helpful, and there are no reliable clinical features to tell us how much 'osis' (wear and tear) and how much 'itis' (inflammation) is contributing to a particular symptomatic joint[40]. Often, the only way to find out is to treat it

- *Breaking up the inflammatory damage–repair–damage cycle*, which is postulated to set up a continuous low-grade inflammatory response, inhibiting tissue repair and sound scar formation, while forming adverse adhesions[41,42]. There is little direct evidence to support this, however

- Possibly a direct *chondroprotective effect* on cartilage metabolism or other effects not related to anti-inflammatory activity of the steroids, e.g. promotion of articular surfactant production[32,43,44,206,216,224–226,241]

Inflammation is a complex cascade of molecular and cellular events that is often poorly understood by the clinicians who treat it[316,317]. The precise role of inflammation in 'tendinitis' is the subject of considerable debate, and many authors prefer the terms 'tendinosis' or 'tendinopathy' to describe the pathological changes[45–48]. The pain might not be due to inflammation (tendinitis) or structural disruption of the tendon fibres (tendinosis), but to the stimulation of nociceptors by chemicals released from the damaged tendon[49]. Corticosteroids (and possibly local anaesthetics) might affect the release of noxious chemicals and/or the long-term behaviour of local nociceptors.

COMMONLY USED CORTICOSTEROIDS (Table 1)

- **Adcortyl**: 10 mg/ml – dilute
- **Kenalog**: 40 mg/ml – concentrated

Triamcinolone acetonide

Throughout the book we recommend Kenalog for ease of administration. This drug can be used in very small quantities and so is ideal for small joints and tendons where distension can increase pain. Adcortyl, however, is useful where larger volume is required as in larger joints and bursae. The duration of action of the drug is approximately 3 weeks[262].

Triamcinolone hexacetonide (Lederspan) was the least soluble and longest-lasting injectable drug available[30,50,193,202] but the manufacturer withdrew it in 2001.

Methylprednisolone acetate

- **Depo-Medrone**: 40 mg/ml – concentrated

This drug may cause more postinjection pain than triamcinalone acetonide[51]. It is also available premixed with local anaesthetic as Depo-Medrone (40 mg/ml) and with lidocaine (10 mg/ml) in 1-ml and 2-ml vials, which we do not recommend because it is a fixed-dose combination and therefore difficult to adjust.

Hydrocortisone

- **Hydrocortistab**: 25 mg/ml – very dilute

Very soluble – this has the shortest duration of action of the steroids mentioned here[52]. We recommend its use particularly for superficial injections in thin, dark-skinned females, where there may be risk of depigmentation or local fat atrophy[53].

Twenty mg of Hydrocortistab is equipotent to 4 mg of triamcinolone or methylprednisolone.

	Drug	Potency	Dose	Manufacturer
	Short-acting	+		
	Hydrocortisone acetate		25 mg/ml	Sovereign
	Hydrocortistab		1-ml ampoules	
	Intermediate-acting	+++++		
	Methylprednisolone acetate		40 mg/ml	Pharmacia
	Depo-Medrone		1-ml, 2-ml,	
			3-ml vials	
	Depo-Medrone + Lidocaine		1-ml, 2-ml vials	
	Tiamcinolone acetonide			Squibb
	Adcortyl		10 mg/ml	
			1-ml ampoules,	
			5-ml vials	
	Kenalog		40 mg/ml	
			1-ml vials	

Table 1
Commonly used
corticosteroids

LOCAL ANAESTHETICS

These membrane-stabilizing drugs act by causing a reversible block to conduction along nerve fibres. The smaller nerve fibres are more sensitive, so that a differential block can occur where the small fibres carrying pain and autonomic impulses are blocked, sparing coarse touch and movement[91]. Following most regional anaesthetic procedures, maximum arterial plasma concentrations of local anaesthetic develop within about 10–25 minutes[91]. This has implications for outpatient practice if significant volumes of the drug are injected.

RATIONALE FOR USING LOCAL ANAESTHETICS

- *Analgesic*: although the effect is temporary, it can make the overall procedure less unpleasant for the patient, break the pain cycle (by reducing nociceptive input to the 'gate' in the dorsal horn of the spinal cord), and increase the confidence of the patient in the clinician, the diagnosis and the treatment. In one study, pain inhibition was better with bupivacaine than lidocaine during the first 6 hours, because of its longer half-life; in later evaluations no differences in outcomes were observed[93]. In another study, bupivacaine was superior to lidocaine at 2 weeks, but not at 3 and 12 months[94]. Some practitioners inject a mixture of short- and long-acting local anaesthetic to obtain both the immediate diagnostic effect plus more prolonged pain relief

- *Diagnostic*: pain relief following an injection confirms the diagnosis and correct placement of the solution[92]. Sometimes even the most experienced practitioner will be unsure exactly which tissue is at fault; in this situation, inject a small amount of local anaesthetic into the most likely tissue, wait a few minutes, and re-examine. If the pain is relieved then the source of the problem has been identified and further treatment can be accurately directed; if not, further testing should follow until sure of the cause of the pain

- *Dilution*: the internal surface area of joints and bursae is surprisingly large, due to the highly convoluted synovial lining with its many villae, so increased volume of the injected solution helps to spread the steroid around this surface

● *Distension*: a beneficial volume effect in joints and bursae might be the stretching of the capsule or bursa with physical disruption of adhesions[95,96,178,217]. Distension is not required at entheses, so use the smallest volume that is practicable; distension in tendons by bolus injection of a relatively large volume of solution may physically disrupt the tendon fibres and compress the relatively poor arterial supply. It can also give rise to distension pain

COMMONLY USED LOCAL ANAESTHETICS

Lidocaine hydrochloride (lignocaine hydrochloride)

The most widely used local anaesthetic, lidocaine hydrochloride acts more rapidly and is more stable than other local anaesthetics. The effect occurs within seconds and duration of block is about half an hour; this is the local anaesthetic we prefer.

Marcain (bupivacaine)

Marcain has a slow onset of action (about 30 minutes for the full effect) but the duration of block can be 8 hours or more. It is the principal drug for spinal anaesthesia in the UK. We do not use it for routine outpatient injections because the delayed onset of action precludes the immediate diagnostic effect available with lidocaine, and if there is an adverse effect it will take a long time to dissipate. There is no evidence of any long-term benefit from using bupivacaine instead of lidocaine[94]. Compared to placebo, the effect of intra-articular bupivacaine wears off in less than 24 hours[228].

Prilocaine and procaine

Prilocaine has low toxicity similar to lidocaine but is not as commonly used. Procaine is now also seldom used; it is as potent as lidocaine but with shorter duration of action.

Lidocaine (under the brand name Xylocaine) and Marcain are also manufactured with added epinephrine (adrenaline) (which causes vasoconstriction when used for skin anaesthesia, and so prolongs the local anaesthetic effect). *Do not* inject these drugs into joints or soft-tissue lesions. Xylocaine is clearly marked in red that it has epinephrine added.

Recommended maximum doses are given in Table 2. In practice, however, we suggest that much lower maximum doses are used (see the section on Injection technique, p 34).

Table 2 Commonly used local anaesthetics with maximum recommended doses (BNF 2006)

Drug	Strength		Maximum dose and volume	
Lidocaine	0.5%	5 mg/ml	200 mg	40 ml
	1.0%	10 mg/ml	200 mg	20 ml
	2.0%	20 mg/ml	200 mg	10 ml
Bupivacaine	0.25%	2.5 mg/ml	150 mg	60 ml
	0.5%	5 mg/ml	150 mg	30 ml

POTENTIAL SIDE-EFFECTS

Side-effects from injection therapy with corticosteroids and/or local anaesthetics are uncommon and, when they do occur, are usually mild and transient[64]. Nonetheless, it is incumbent upon the clinician practising injection therapy to be aware of the presentation and management of all the potential minor and more serious side-effects associated with this treatment[5].

Consider carefully before giving corticosteroid injections to pregnant or breastfeeding women; this treatment is often recommended for carpal tunnel syndrome and de Quervain's tenovaginitis[62,239]. There is no evidence that the woman or her baby will be harmed[181] – indeed, cortisol levels rise in pregnancy – but pregnancy and childbirth are highly emotive and if the mother has a difficult delivery or a baby with an abnormality she might try to blame the injection. Detailed discussion of the benefits and potential adverse effects of injection therapy should be carefully documented.

LOCAL SIDE-EFFECTS

Most local side-effects occur when too large a dose, in too large a volume, is injected too often. Subcutaneous placement of the steroid and using a bolus technique at the entheses of tendons must be avoided.

Postinjection flare of pain

The quoted figures are from about 2% to 10%[63,64], but this is well in excess of our own experience. When it does happen it is usually after a soft-tissue injection, and rarely follows joint injection[64]. It appears to be caused by rapid intracellular ingestion of the microcrystalline steroid ester and must always be distinguished from sepsis[28,31,36,260]. There appear to be more frequent postinjection flares with methylprednisolone but this might have more to do with the preservative in the drug than with the steroid itself[57]. An early increase in joint stiffness following intra-articular corticosteroids is consistent with a transient synovitis[179].

Multidose bottles of lidocaine (Xylocaine) contain parabens as a preservative. Many steroids will precipitate when added to parabens and this precipitate might be responsible for some cases of postinjection flare of pain and 'steroid chalk' (see below). Parabens might also be responsible for some allergic reactions to local injections. The use of multidose bottles increases the risk of cross-infection and should be avoided[220]. Single-dose vials of lidocaine do not contain parabens.

Subcutaneous atrophy and/or skin depigmentation[31,65]

This is more likely to occur when superficial lesions are injected, especially in dark-skinned patients[53,66]. Take care not to allow injected drugs to reflux back through the needle tract – pressure around the needle with cotton wool when withdrawing can help. In thin dark-skinned women especially, it might be preferable to use hydrocortisone for superficial lesions. These patients must always be advised of the possibility of this side-effect, and the fact recorded in the notes. Local atrophy appears within 1–4 months of injection and characteristically proceeds to resolution 6–24 months later, but may take longer[263].

Bleeding or bruising

These can occur at the injection site, especially in patients taking warfarin, aspirin or NSAIDs with significant antiplatelet activity, e.g. naproxen.

Steroid 'chalk' or 'paste'

This might be found on the surface of previously injected tendons and joints during surgery. Suspension flocculation, resulting from the mixture of steroid with a local anaesthetic containing preservative, might be responsible. The clinical significance of these deposits is uncertain[31].

Soft-tissue calcification Corticosteroid injections into osteoarthritic interphalangeal joints of the hand can result in calcification or joint fusion, possibly because of pericapsular leakage of steroids due to raised intra-articular pressure[68]. No deleterious effects have been ascribed to this calcification.

Steroid arthropathy This is a well known and much feared complication of local injection treatment – it is also largely a myth[69]. There is evidence that in many instances injected steroids can be chondroprotective rather than destructive[31,43], but the information from animal models about whether steroids damage or protect joints is contradictory[70,184]. There is good evidence linking prolonged high-dose *oral* steroid usage with osteonecrosis, but almost all the reports linking injected steroids with accelerated non-septic joint destruction are anecdotal, and mainly relate to joints receiving huge numbers of injections[69]. A reasonable guide[71] is to give injections into the major joints in the lower limbs at no less than 3-month intervals, although this advice is based on consensus rather than evidence[72,185]. Reports of Charcot-like accelerated joint destruction after corticosteroid injection in human hip osteoarthritis (OA) might reflect the disease itself rather than the treatment[31,73]. Currently, no evidence supports the promotion of disease progression by steroid injections[164,192]. Repeat injections into the knee joint every 3 months seem to be safe over 2 years[165].

Tendon rupture[74–77,166] or atrophy[78] These are probably minimized by careful attention to technique, i.e. withdraw the needle a little if an unusual amount of resistance is encountered[74], and use a peppering technique at the enthesis with the smallest effective dose and volume of steroid[79]. The whole issue of steroid-associated tendon rupture is controversial[19,20,75–77,167], disputed[80], anecdotal[74,169] and – in humans – is not well supported in the literature[2,76], although it is widely accepted that the repeated injection of steroids into load-bearing tendons carries the risk of tendon rupture[81].

The current climate of opinion among consultants in locomotor specialties is equivocal about steroid injection around the Achilles tendon. If this is being contemplated it is advisable to image the tendon first (by MRI or ultrasound) to confirm that it is a peritendinitis with no tendinopathy (degenerative change with or without tears in the body of the tendon). Low-dose peritendinous steroid injections appear to be safe[161]. The patient should rest from provocative activity for 6–8 weeks[75] (consider putting the keen athlete into a walking cast), and return to it gradually after a graduated programme of stretching and strengthening. In rabbits, local injections of corticosteroid, both within the tendon substance and into the retrocalcaneal bursa, adversely affect the biomechanical properties of Achilles tendons. Additionally, tendons from rabbits that have received bilateral injections of corticosteroid demonstrate significantly worse biomechanical properties than tendons from those that have received unilateral injections of corticosteroid. Bilateral injections of corticosteroids should be avoided because they might impart a systemic effect in conjunction with the local effect, further weakening the tendon[143]. Surgery for chronic Achilles tendinopathy has a complication rate of around 10% and should not be assumed to be a trouble-free treatment option[168].

Joint sepsis[82] This is the most feared complication of steroid injection treatment. It can be lethal[243] but it is a rarity, occurring in only one in 17,000–77,000 patients when performed as an 'office' procedure[31,68,83,84]. Soft-tissue infections and osteomyelitis can also occur after local soft tissue injection[203,209]. Prompt recognition of infection is essential to prevent joint and soft tissue destruction, and diagnosis can be delayed by mistaking joint sepsis for postinjection flare or exacerbation of the underlying arthropathy[85]. Swelling at the injection site, increased pain, fever, systemic upset (e.g. sweating, headaches) and dysfunction of the affected part following a local injection should all raise clinical suspicion of infection. A case report by the Medical Defence Union highlighted a patient who developed septic arthritis following a steroid injection into the shoulder joint by her general practitioner. The opinion of two experts was that infection is a rare hazard of the procedure, for which the GP should not be blamed, but that failure to recognize and appropriately manage this side effect is difficult to defend[86].

Fragments of skin can be carried into a joint on the tip of a needle and might be a source of infection[268]. Joint infections might also occur by haematogenous spread, rather than by direct inoculation of organisms into the joint. Steroid injection can create a local focus of reduced immunity in a joint, thus rendering it more vulnerable to blood-borne spread from a distant infected site, e.g. urinary tract or chest infection. Rarely, injection of contaminated drugs or hormonal activation of a quiescent infection may be to blame[82,85].

All cases of suspected infection following injection must be promptly admitted to hospital for diagnosis and treatment[82]. Blood tests (ESR, CRP, plasma viscosity, white blood cell differential count, blood cultures) should be taken, along with diagnostic aspiration of the affected joint or any other localized swelling. The needle used for attempted aspiration can be sent for culture if no aspirate is obtained[203]. X-ray changes might be absent in the early stages of joint infection and more sophisticated imaging techniques, such as MRI and isotope bone scans, might be helpful.

To avoid injecting an already infected joint, have a high index of suspicion in patients with RA[87], elderly OA patients with an acute monarthritic flare (especially hip) and patients with coexistent infection elsewhere, e.g. chest, urinary tract, skin (especially the legs). Visualize and dipstick the urine and check the ESR[88].

In the largest series of bacterial isolates reported from UK patients with septic arthritis, the most common organisms were *Staphylococcus aureus* and streptococci species. Others were *Escherichia coli*, *Haemophilus influenzae*, *Salmonella* species, *Pseudomonas* species and *Mycobacterium tuberculosis*[89]. *M. tuberculosis* can be particularly difficult to diagnose and might require the study of synovial biopsy samples[85]. Infection was most common in children and the elderly. Underlying risk factors were reported in one-fifth of cases, the most frequent being a prosthetic joint (11%). Others included haematological malignancy, joint disease or connective-tissue disorder, diabetes, oral steroid therapy, chemotherapy, presence of an intravenous line, intravenous drug abuse and postarthroscopy[89]. Some surgeons deprecate the routine use of intra-articular steroids following arthroscopy for OA knee because of a perceived increased risk of infection following this procedure[70]. Steroid injection can also delay the presentation of sepsis by 6–12 days[70].

Joint infection has been reported as occurring between 4 days and 3 weeks after injection[203]. Exotic infections might occur in immunocompromised patients following joint injection[219].

Aggressive therapy, including cytotoxic drugs, is increasingly used in the treatment of rheumatoid arthritis (RA) and might confer increased susceptibility to infections. Septic arthritis is one infectious complication known to be over-represented in RA. In one small series of RA patients with septic arthritis, six out of nine had received an intra-articular injection into the infected joint within 3 months prior to the onset of the sepsis; only one of these occurred immediately after joint injection. The annual frequency of septic arthritis was approximately 0.2%; during the 4-year period studied the frequency was 0.5%. When related to the number of steroid injections, a frequency of 1 per 2000 injections was found when late septic arthritis was included. The high frequency of delayed septic arthritis in RA patients after intra-articular steroid administration should alert clinicians to this complication[214].

If a local infection occurs following an injection, vigorous attempts must be made to isolate the causative organism. If this is *Staphylococcus aureus*, the clinician should have personal nasal swabs taken. If these confirm nasal carriage of this organism, the clinician should receive appropriate antibiotic treatment and not give any more injections until further swabs confirm clearance of the organism. A review of the aseptic technique used should also be undertaken[203].

Intra-articular corticosteroids can be effective following septic arthritis when pain and synovitis persist despite adequate intravenous antibiotic treatment, and where lavage and repeat synovial fluid and blood cultures are found to be sterile[196]. The use of corticosteroid pre-packaged in a sterile syringe may reduce the risk of infection[84]. Multidose bottles and vials should be avoided because they can become contaminated and act as a source of infection[220]. Drugs for injection must be stored in accordance with the manufacturer's instructions.

Rare local side-effects

These include:

- *Nerve damage*: severe pain and 'electric shocks' if you needle a nerve

- *Transient paresis of an extremity*: from an inadvertent motor nerve block

- *Needle fracture*[5,31,34,67]

- *Delayed soft-tissue healing* can be associated with local steroid injection. In a study of rabbit ligaments, the tensile strength of the specimens that had been injected with the steroids returned to a value that was equal to that of the controls that had not received an injection; however, the peak load of the specimens that had been injected with steroids remained inferior to that of the controls. This was accompanied by a lag in the histological maturation[176]. This has implications for the timing of return to activity, especially sport, following injection therapy

- *Injection of the wrong drug* is a potentially serious and totally avoidable problem with severe consequences for all concerned[67]. Strict attention to the preparation protocol should prevent this

In a large prospective study carried out in an orthopaedic outpatient department, complications of injection therapy were recorded in 672 patients receiving 1147 injections[64]. Just under 12% of patients (7% of injections) had any side-effect, but almost all of these were transient. Only four patients had subcutaneous atrophy at the injection site and these were all tennis elbow injections in females; the steroid dose was 4 times the dose we recommend. The commonest side-effect was post-injection pain, but methylprednisolone was used which we believe causes more pain when injected into soft tissues than triamcinolone. When the data are reanalysed, 12% of the patients receiving periarticular injections had postinjection pain, but only 2% of those with intra-articular injections. Other side effects were bleeding and fainting or dizziness.

Injection therapy for joints and soft tissues is a very safe form of treatment. Compared with the safety profile of oral non-steroidal anti-inflammatory drugs, the justification for using the minimum effective dose of injectable drugs in the correct place with appropriate preparation and aftercare becomes evident[90] (Table 3).

Table 3 Numbers needed to harm for patients >60 prescribed oral NSAIDs >2 months (from Tramer et al[90])	Number	Harm caused
	1 in 5	Endoscopic ulcer
	1 in 70	Symptomatic ulcer
	1 in 150	Bleeding ulcer
	1 in 1200	Death from bleeding ulcer

SYSTEMIC SIDE-EFFECTS (Table 4)

Facial flushing[36]
Probably the most common side-effect, occurring in from 5% of patients[1] to less than 1%[31]. It can come on within 24–48 hours after the injection and lasts 1–2 days.

Impaired diabetic control[242]
Diabetic patients must be warned about this possible temporary side effect. A common observation is that blood sugar levels undergo a modest rise for up to a week, rarely longer. This might occasionally require a short-term increase in diabetic drug dosage, so the patient should be informed about the steroid drug and dosage given.

Menstrual irregularity (pre- and postmenopausal)[4,54]
The mechanism is unknown (ovulation might be inhibited)[34]. In a postmenopausal woman this then creates a difficult dilemma – is the bleeding related to the injection or should she be investigated to exclude other, potentially serious, causes of postmenopausal bleeding? If this complication occurs it must always be taken seriously.

Hypothalamic–pituitary axis suppression[55]
Occurs following intra-articular and intramuscular injection of corticosteroids[31,56,183], but at the doses and frequencies used in our approach to injection therapy this appears to be of no significant clinical consequence[57]

therefore we do not issue patients with a steroid card after injection[182]. Greater systemic absorption occurs if a steroid is injected into several joints, presumably due to the greater synovial surface area available for drug transfer[31,183]. Peak plasma levels of prednisolone acetate occur 2–4 hours after injection into the rheumatoid knee[190]. This accounts for the common observation of symptomatic improvement in joints other than the one injected.

Significant fall in ESR and CRP levels (mean fall of about 50%) Intraarticular corticosteroid injections can cause this in patients with inflammatory arthritis and this effect can last for up to 6 months. This needs to be taken into account when using these blood tests to assess the response of patients to disease-modifying drugs like Salazopyrin and methotrexate[58].

Anaphylaxis Severe anaphylactic reactions to local anaesthetic injections are rare, but can be fatal[59-61]. Anaphylactic reactions to locally injected corticosteroids are very rare but can occur[1]. They might be a reaction to the stabilizers the drug is mixed with rather than the steroid drug itself[57].

Other rare systemic side-effects from local steroid injection treatment include *pancreatitis* (patient presents with abdominal pain and the serum amylase is raised), *nausea*, *dysphoria* (emotional upset), *acute psychosis*, *myopathy* and *posterior subcapsular cataracts*[5,31,34,180,211].

Table 4 Potential side-effects of corticosteroid/ local anaesthetic injection therapy

Systemic side-effects	Local side-effects
Facial flushing	Postinjection flare of pain
Impaired diabetic control	Skin depigmentation, fat atrophy
Menstrual irregularity	Bleeding/bruising
Hypothalamic–pituitary axis suppression	Steroid 'chalk', calcification
Fall in ESR/CRP	Steroid arthropathy
Anaphylaxis	Tendon rupture/atrophy
	Joint/soft-tissue sepsis

OTHER INJECTABLE SUBSTANCES

EPINEPHRINE (ADRENALINE) Epinephrine is a vasoconstrictor, which acts on the noradrenaline receptors and immediately physiologically reverses the symptoms of bronchospasm, laryngeal oedema and hypotension occurring in anaphylaxis or angioedema[97].

Epinephrine should always be at hand when using injection therapy in case of an anaphylactic reaction to the local anaesthetic. This may be conveniently carried in the form of an EpiPen, which is an autoinjector for intramuscular use, preloaded with 1 mg/ml of epinephrine and delivering a single dose of 0.3 ml (epinephrine 1 : 1000)[59-61].

SCLEROSANTS Sclerotherapy[41,291] aims to strengthen inadequate ligaments by injecting them with an irritant to induce fibroblast hyperplasia; this causes soft-tissue inflammation, the opposite of steroid therapy. In the USA this treatment is known as prolotherapy because it involves injecting a proliferant – a substance that causes fibroblast proliferation.

Sclerosing therapy was used by Hippocrates in the form of cautery at the shoulder to prevent recurrent shoulder dislocation. It is mainly used to treat varicose veins, oesophageal varices and piles; its use in locomotor disorders is not widespread. It is mostly used in back lesions but might also be indicated for peripheral instability.

There are a large number of sclerosants, a common one being P2G, which contains phenol, glucose and glycerine. Some prefer to use dextrose, which is potentially less neurotoxic, although part of the pain-relieving effect might be due to a toxic action on nociceptors. Sclerosants are usually diluted with a local anaesthetic.

In the most carefully conducted study of the use of sclerosants in back pain so far carried out, there was no difference between the effect of injecting a sclerosant solution or injecting saline at key spinal ligament entheses; but, as both groups of patients improved significantly, it is difficult to decide what the particular effect of sclerosant injections might be[230].

Long-term effects of intra-articular dextrose sclerotherapy for anterior cruciate ligament laxity have been reported as favourable in a small study[229]. The anecdotal experience of the authors is that this treatment might be worth trying in conditions where the symptoms are caused by chronic ligamentous laxity, e.g. at the ankle, thumb or sacroiliac joint, or where other conservative interventions have failed.

A pilot study has reported an intriguing new use for sclerosants in the treatment of tendinopathy. Neovascularization (new blood vessel formation) occurs in Achilles tendinopathy. Polidocanol, a sclerosing local anaesthetic, was injected into the neovessels under colour Doppler ultrasound control. Eight out of ten subjects had a significant reduction in their pain and returned to pain-free tendon loading activities with benefit persisting at 6 months[292]. Larger longer-term double-blind randomized controlled trials of this approach are eagerly awaited. It would be especially useful to know how a 'blind' approach compares to injection using ultrasound guidance.

LUBRICANTS In osteoarthritic joints, the capacity of synovial fluid to lubricate and absorb shock is typically reduced. This is partly due to a reduction in the size and concentration of hyaluronic acid (hyaluronan) molecules naturally present in synovial fluid. These molecules produce a highly viscoelastic solution that is a viscous lubricant at low shear (during slow movement of the joint, as in walking) and an elastic shock absorber at high shear (during rapid movement, as in running). Hyaluronic acid is considered not only a joint lubricant but also a physiological factor in the trophic status of cartilage. It has a very high water-binding capacity; when 1 g of hyaluronic acid is dissolved in physiological saline, it occupies 3 litres of solution[222]. Osteoarthritis of the knee can be treated by the intra-articular injection of hyaluronan or its derivatives (hylan)[100,208], usually after any effusion is drained. This treatment option is endorsed by two authoritative guidelines[173,174]. The mode of action of exogenous hyaluronan and its derivatives is not clear; they stay in the joint cavity for only a few days. Perhaps they stimulate endogenous hyaluronan synthesis and/or reduce inflammation.

The licensed commercial formulations which have been available the longest in the UK are Hyalgan and Synvisc, but there is no evidence that one is superior[175]. Hyalgan has the lower molecular weight of the two and is licensed as a medicinal product. It is injected once weekly for 5 weeks and is repeatable no more than 6 monthly. Synvisc has a higher molecular weight and is licensed as a medical device. It is injected once weekly for 3 weeks, repeatable once within 6 months, with at least 4 weeks between courses. Compared to placebo, both products produce a small reduction in pain that can last several months[201]. The limited data available suggest that the products are as effective as continuous treatment with oral NSAIDs or intra-articular corticosteroid injections[100], but at significantly greater cost.

Intra-articular injection of hyaluronic acid can decrease symptoms of osteoarthritis of the knee, with significant improvements in pain and functional outcomes and few adverse events[172,213]. They might cause a short-term increase in knee inflammation[175,177]. Studies of lower methodological quality, such as a single-blind or single-centre design indicate higher estimates of efficacy. Patients older than 65 and those with the most advanced radiographic stage of osteoarthritis (complete loss of the joint space) are less likely to benefit[172].

Synvisc is licensed for use in the hip joint. The use of lubricant injections in other joints is being investigated[221,236,237].

One study used a combination of Hyalgan and corticosteroid injections initially. The corticosteroid injections seemed to increase the long-term efficacy of the hyaluronic acid, suggesting that the combination of these two local treatments would be a promising approach to therapy. More research is needed[227].

Many other substances including NSAIDs[222], morphine[157], methotrexate[158], guanethidine[101], radioactive materials[34,102], anakinra (an interleukin-1 receptor antagonist)[156], osmic acid (for chemical synovectomy[200]) and even air[95,96] have been injected into joints to investigate their therapeutic potential. None can currently be recommended for routine administration.

DRUG NAMES

In the past, some drugs have gone under different generic names in different countries. In 1992 the European Community decreed that all member countries should use the World Health Organization's recommended international non-proprietary name (RINN). In the UK, lignocaine has been changed to lidocaine and adrenaline is now epinephrine (with dual labelling to avoid confusion in emergencies)[103].

COSTS

All of the injectable drugs we use are remarkably inexpensive (UK prices 2005) (Table 5).

Compare the costs of injectable drugs with the cost of some commonly prescribed oral NSAIDs (Table 6).

Injection therapy is also cost-effective when compared to conventional physiotherapy[105].

Table 5	Injectable drugs 2005	Cost
The costs of some injectable drugs	1-ml ampoule Adcortyl (10 mg of triamcinolone acetonide)	£1.02
	1-ml vial Kenalog (40 mg)	£1.70
	10 ml 1% lidocaine	£0.35

Table 6	NSAIDs 2005	Cost
Costs of common oral NSAIDs	Generic ibuprofen – 1 month at 400 mg tds	£2.74
	Generic diclofenac – 1 month at 50 mg tds	£1.45
	Voltarol – 1 month at 50 mg tds	£5.71[97]

SECTION 1

SAFETY

ASEPTIC TECHNIQUE

The following simple precautions should be taken to prevent occurrence of sepsis:

- Remove watches and jewellery
- Mark the injection site with the closed end of a sterile needle guard, then discard
- Clean the injection site with appropriate cleanser and allow 1 min to dry[104, 204]
- Wash hands thoroughly for 1 min; dry well on disposable paper towel*
- Use prepacked, in-date, sterile, disposable needles and syringes
- Use single-dose ampoules or vials, then discard
- Change needles after drawing-up the solution into the syringe
- Do not touch the skin after marking and cleansing the site
- Do not guide the needle with a finger
- When injecting a joint, aspirate to check that any fluid found does not look infected

Remember: wet hands carry an increased risk of infection[104, 106–109], so hands must be well dried before injecting.

In some countries gloves are mandatory[110, 111]. We recommend the use of gloves when aspirating or when sepsis is suspected[9]. Scrubbing up or wearing of gowns is not normally required.

IMMEDIATE ADVERSE REACTIONS

The most important immediate adverse reactions to injection therapy are:

- acute anaphylaxis
- toxicity from local anaesthetic
- syncope

ACUTE ANAPHYLAXIS

Acute systemic anaphylaxis results from widespread mast cell degranulation triggered by a specific allergen. Clinically, it is characterized by laryngeal oedema, bronchospasm and hypotension[144]. The true incidence of anaphylaxis is unknown. Fatal anaphylaxis is rare but probably underestimated. A register established in 1992 recording fatal reactions gave an incidence of only 20 cases a year in the UK, of which half were iatrogenic, mainly occurring in hospital, a quarter were related to food allergy, and a quarter were related to venom allergy[145].

Hypersensitivity to local anaesthetic occurs very rarely[91, 112] and mainly with the ester-types, e.g. procaine, and less frequently with the amide types, e.g. lidocaine and bupivacaine[91]. A patient can be allergic to local anaesthetic and be unaware of it. A previous uneventful injection is not a guarantee that the patient will not be allergic this time, although it does provide some reassurance. The features might be any of those listed in Table 7[113]. Circulatory collapse, cardiac arrest and death might follow.

Table 7 The symptoms and signs of acute anaphylaxis	Symptoms	Signs
	Nervousness	Skin changes; flushing/ pallor/cyanosis/ urticaria
	Itchy skin	
	Feeling of impending catastrophe	Laryngeal oedema, stridor, angio-oedema
	Feeling drunk or confused	Tachycardia
	Nausea, vomiting, diarrhoea	Profound hypotension/decreased capillary filling
	Abdominal or back pain	
	Rhinitis/conjunctivitis	Convulsions
		Respiratory depression
		Bronchospasm/severe respiratory difficulty

TOXICITY FROM LOCAL ANAESTHETIC

Toxic effects from local anaesthetic are usually a result of excessive plasma concentrations. Care must be taken to avoid accidental intravascular injection. The main toxic effects are excitation of the CNS followed by CNS depression (Table 8). Hypersensitivity to local anaesthetic occurs very rarely[91, 112].

With intravenous injection, convulsions and cardiovascular collapse can occur very rapidly.

Table 8 Toxic effects from local anaesthetics	Symptoms	Signs
	Lightheadedness	Sedation
	Feeling drunk	Circumoral paraesthesia, twitching
		Convulsions in severe reactions

SYNCOPE

A few people might faint not as a reaction to *what* was injected but to *being* injected – the result of pain or needle phobia. Patients who express apprehension before having an injection should lie down for the procedure. The clinician might be so intent on placing the needle correctly that the warning features are missed.

Syncope must be distinguished from an adverse drug reaction, and is treated by:

- reassuring the patient that he or she will shortly recover
- lying the patient down in the recovery position
- if loss of consciousness occurs, protecting the airway and giving 35% oxygen

Syncope might be accompanied by brief jerking or stiffening of the extremities and can be mistaken for a convulsion by the inexperienced. Distinguishing a simple faint from a fit is helped by the presence of precipitating factors (painful stimuli, fear), and the other features described above. Incontinence is rare with syncope and recovery of consciousness usually occurs within 1 minute[114].

<table>
<tr><td>Table 9
The symptoms and signs of syncope</td><td>Symptoms</td><td>Signs</td></tr>
<tr><td></td><td>Lightheadedness, dizziness
Tell you they are going to faint
Nausea
Ringing in the ears
Vision 'going grey'</td><td>Pallor
Sweating
Slight swaying
Bradycardia
Hypotension</td></tr>
</table>

TREATMENT OF SEVERE ALLERGIC REACTIONS

Clinicians will give injections in a variety of settings, including in hospital, with and without a 'crash' team, and in various community premises, including primary care and private facilities. Clinicians must prepare for the 'worst-case scenario' in their setting and have a well thought-out plan of action that is regularly reviewed in the light of current guidelines and individual experience. Basic life-support skills should be acquired and maintained. Written protocols should be laminated and mounted in consulting rooms.

Immediate action in the presence of signs of severe anaphylaxis, i.e. clinical signs of shock, hypotension, airway swelling or definite breathing difficulties:

- Stop injecting
- Lie the patient flat, if breathing permits
- Maintain airway
- Summon help
- Administer 500 micrograms (0.5 ml 1:1000) epinephrine (adrenaline) or EpiPen intramuscularly
- Administer oxygen if necessary
- Give cardiopulmonary resuscitation if necessary
- Administer Piriton or hydrocortisone if required
- Transfer the patient to hospital as quickly as possible if the reaction occurs in the community

For further details on the current guideline for the management of anaphylaxis, see Resuscitation Council advice and algorithms 2002 at: www.resus.org.uk.

ADVERSE REACTION REPORTING

In the UK, all severe adverse reactions to any drug treatment should be reported to the Committee on Safety of Medicines (CSM) using the Yellow Card system. Yellow Card report forms can be found in the back of the *British National Formulary* (BNF).

PREVENTION OF ADVERSE REACTIONS

Clinicians must be prepared for any adverse reaction. Take the following precautions:

- Ask patients about any known allergies to drugs, especially local anaesthetics, e.g. an allergic reaction to a dental injection
- If in doubt, give an injection of steroid alone or steroid diluted with normal saline
- Give the injection with the patient lying down
- Control the amount of local anaesthetic given (see Injection Technique Guidelines, p. 33)
- Always aspirate before injecting, to check that the needle is not in a blood vessel
- Ask the patient to wait in the surgery for 30 minutes after the injection

Anaphylactic reactions begin rapidly, usually within 5–10 minutes of exposure. The time taken for full reaction to evolve varies, but is usually 10–30 minutes[113]. Occasionally, a delayed reaction occurs after a few hours.

Epinephrine reverses the immediate symptoms of anaphylaxis by its effects on alpha and beta adrenoceptors. It reverses peripheral vasodilatation, reduces oedema, induces bronchodilatation, has positive inotropic and chronotropic effects on the myocardium, and suppresses further mediator release. It can be harmful if given outside of the context of life-threatening anaphylaxis[144].

Preloaded devices such as EpiPen, which delivers 300 micrograms of epinephrine, can be used in the home or community. Although this is less than the recommended dose of 500 micrograms for adults, this may be sufficient. The dose should be repeated 5 minutes after the first dose *only if* the patient continues to deteriorate.

In a series of deaths related to anaphylaxis, two deaths occurred after epinephrine overdose in the absence of anaphylaxis, three deaths occurred after epinephrine overdose in the context of allergic reactions, and two fatal myocardial infarctions occurred after epinephrine administration for mild iatrogenic reactions (where less aggressive treatment might have been appropriate)[145]. Administering the doses recommended in the guidelines via the *intramuscular* route should avoid serious problems.

HEALTH AND SAFETY

Clinicians should be vaccinated against hepatitis B and have had a blood test to confirm immunity[115]. A booster vaccination every 5 years might be necessary. If in doubt, a doctor or hospital occupational health department specialist should be consulted.

Local policies on needle-stick injuries must be observed: there are national guidelines on the occupational exposure to HIV[116,117]. The best way to avoid a needle-stick injury is to be well organized and never to rush an injection.

EMERGENCY SUPPLIES FOR THE TREATMENT ROOM

Have a supply of emergency equipment and medication available.

ESSENTIAL EMERGENCY KIT
- Disposable plastic airways
- An ambubag and mask for assisted ventilation
- Epinephrine 1 : 1000 strength or EpiPen
- Oxygen with masks and tubing

ADDITIONAL EMERGENCY KIT FOR MEDICAL PERSONNEL
- Chlorphenamine (Piriton) for injection
- Hydrocortisone for injection
- Nebulized salbutamol
- A selection of intravenous cannulae and fluid-giving sets
- Normal saline for infusion
- Plasma substitute for infusion

All drugs and fluids should be checked regularly to ensure they are in date.

DRUGS AND SPORT

Under the International Olympic Committee Medical Commission list of Prohibited Substances and Methods (2004), local anaesthetics are permitted (except for cocaine)[186]. In competition, corticosteroids come under the heading of 'Prohibited Substances and Methods' section S9 when administered orally, rectally or by intravenous or intramuscular injection. All other routes of administration (e.g. intra-articular) require the submission of a Therapeutic Use Exemptions (TUE) form to the appropriate authorities[186]. Corticosteroids are not banned outside competition[188] but athletes are warned that they are subject to the rule of strict liability, which means that they are responsible for any prohibited substance found in their body. It is each athlete's personal duty to ensure that no prohibited substance enters his or her body. Athletes are also responsible for any prohibited substance or its metabolites or markers found present in their bodily specimens.

Accordingly, it is not necessary that intent, fault, negligence or knowing use on the athlete's part be demonstrated to establish an anti-doping violation under article 2.1 of the International Olympic Committee anti-doping rules[187]. It is expected that most athletes competing in the Olympic Games who require a TUE would have already received it from their International Federation. Under the World Anti-doping Agency (WADA) Code, corticosteroids are one of a number of specified substances which are particularly susceptible to unintentional anti-doping rule violations because of their general availability in medicinal products[188].

Doctors and athletes should, however, seek specific advice about drug restrictions with their own sport's governing body. For example, in the UK the Football Association (FA) Doping Control Programme Regulations (2004–5) list local anaesthetics and glucocorticosteroids in class III 'Classes of Drugs Subject to Certain Restrictions'. Local or intra-articular injections of local anaesthetics (excluding cocaine) and glucocorticosteroids are permitted only when medically justified, i.e. the diagnosis, dose and route of administration must have been submitted immediately in writing to the Administator of the FA Doping Control Unit[189]. Compare this with the anti-doping regulations in rugby union, which flow down from WADA to the International Rugby Board (IRB) and then on to the member unions including the Rugby Football Union (RFU). Exactly whose rules and regulations apply at any specific time depends on whose behalf the test is being carried out. There is sufficient internal consistency between the three sets of regulations for them to be effectively the same regarding local and intra-articular steroids (although with some minor differences in wording) but they do differ substantially with respect to local anaesthetics. These cannot be used on match days except in the treatment of bleeding wounds, dental lesions and medical emergencies, i.e. they cannot be used as local anaesthetics pre-game. At this time they are not prohibited under the WADA Code but their use is expressly forbidden under the IRB medical regulations (Dr Simon Kemp, the RFU, personal communication).

If you are not the team doctor and wish to use injection therapy for an athlete, we recommend that you discuss this with the team doctor. The athlete should be provided with a letter describing the rationale for treatment and the names and doses of drugs prescribed. If selected for a drugs test, the athlete should declare the treatment on the doping control form. Virtually insoluble corticosteroids can be detectable months after the injection, although just how many months is difficult to say.

The use of local anaesthetic injections to temporarily block pain and allow athletes to compete while carrying a painful injury is a contentious issue. Clinicians looking after players who request such interventions are recommended to read Orchard's balanced, detailed and pragmatic description of his experience in Australian professional football. His conclusion is that local anaesthetic for pain relief can be used for certain injuries, although complications can be expected. The use of local anaesthetic in professional football can reduce the number of players missing matches through injury but there is the risk of worsening the injury, which should be fully explained to players. A procedure should be used only when both the doctor and player consider that the benefits outweigh the risks[238,264].

Beware athletes who are taking performance-enhancing drugs. They will probably not admit it, but if they develop complications from the use of anabolic steroids, for example, they might blame your injection. Look out for the very muscular athlete with bad skin. Otherwise healthy people, especially those who seem excessively dedicated to developing their physique, need to be asked specifically about their use of illicit drugs[259].

Detailed reviews of the use of injection therapy[39,170] and drug abuse in sport[81,188,259] can be found elsewhere. UK Sport's Drug Information Database provides accurate and timely responses to queries about the status of licensed pharmaceutical products and over-the-counter medicinal products available in the UK in relation to the Olympic Movement Anti-Doping Code. Full details can be found at: www.uksport.gov.uk/did.

MEDICOLEGAL CONSIDERATIONS

CONSENT   The courts require information to be disclosed to the patient in a discussion with the clinician. Thus simply handing patients an explicit consent form might not be considered sufficient unless the issues are discussed with patients and they have an opportunity to ask further questions[293].

INJECTION THERAPY BY HEALTH PROFESSIONALS OTHER THAN DOCTORS   In 1995, the Chartered Society of Physiotherapy (CSP) brought injection therapy into the remit of appropriately trained chartered physiotherapists in the UK. It is now commonly used in hospital outpatient departments, community settings and in private practice. The NHS Plan (2000) envisaged the breaking down of professional barriers and the extension of prescribing rights to health professionals other than doctors[142]. Training in supplementary prescribing for chartered physiotherapists has now been approved (2005).

The most recent advice from The Medical Defence Union (1999) is that a doctor delegating a task or referring a patient should ensure that the person to whom they are delegating or referring is competent[21] and is registered with a statutory regulatory body. Chartered physiotherapists working outside the NHS are personally liable for any claims arising out of their negligent acts or omissions and may require personal indemnity, while those working within the NHS are indemnified by their employer.

PATIENT GROUP DIRECTION (PGD)   In the UK, recent changes to the Medicines Act (1968) allow doctors to sign patient group directions. These allow other clinicians to administer medicines to groups of patients rather than named individuals. According to the Medicines Control Agency, to be lawful (from 9 August 2000), a group protocol should include:

- the signature of a doctor
- signature by representative of appropriate health organization
- the name of business to which the direction applies
- the dates the direction comes into force and expires
- a description of the medicines to which the direction applies
- clinical conditions or situations to which the direction applies
- clinical criteria under which the patient is eligible for treatment
- exclusions from treatment under the direction
- the class of health professional who can supply or administer the medicines
- circumstances in which further advice should be sought from a doctor
- details of maximum dose, quantity, pharmaceutical form and strength, route of administration, frequency and duration of administration
- relevant warnings
- details of any necessary follow-up action
- arrangements for referral for medical advice
- a statement for records to be kept for audit arrangements

A PGD proforma to aid chartered physiotherapists wishing to supply or administer drugs to patients can be obtained from: Stephanie Saunders FCSP, 20 Ailsa Road, Twickenham TW1 1QW, UK. E-mail: stephanie.saunders@virgin.net.

USE OF DRUGS BEYOND LICENCE

This section is adapted from *The use of drugs beyond licence in palliative care and pain management*; recommendations of the Association for Palliative Medicine and The Pain Society. The following statement should be seen as reflecting the views of a responsible body of opinion within these clinical specialties. The full document can be found at: www.rcoa.ac.uk.

The Medicines Control Agency in the UK grants a product licence for a medical drug. The purpose of the licence is to regulate the activity of the pharmaceutical company when marketing the drug; this does not restrict the prescription of the drug by properly qualified medical practitioners.

Licensed drugs can be used legally in clinical situations that fall outside the remit of the licence (referred to as 'off-label'), for example a different age group, a different indication, a different dose or route or method of administration. Sometimes off-label drugs are used because manufacturers have not sought to extend the terms of the licence for economic reasons, where costs are likely to exceed financial return. Use of unlicensed drugs refers to those products that have no licence for any clinical situation or may be in the process of evaluation leading to such a licence.

Injection therapy can involve the use of unlicensed drugs, e.g. sclerosants; 'off label' drugs, e.g. Kenalog (triamcinolone acetonide), which is not licensed to be mixed with lidocaine; and lidocaine, which is not specifically licensed for intra-articular injection, although it *is* licensed for surface infiltration and the caudal route.

From an organizational perspective, the risks presented to clinicians when using drugs beyond licence are best managed through a culture of clinical governance. Organizations should encourage staff to educate themselves and take responsibility for their own decisions within the framework of a corporate policy. There should be mechanisms in place to inform, change and monitor clinical practice:

- The use of drugs beyond licence should be seen as a legitimate aspect of clinical practice
- The use of drugs beyond licence in pain management practice is currently both necessary and common
- Choice of treatment requires partnership between patients and healthcare professionals, and informed consent should be obtained, whenever possible, before prescribing any drug
- Patients should be informed of any identifiable risks and details of any information given should be recorded. It is often unnecessary to take additional steps when recommending drugs beyond licence
- Health professionals involved in prescribing, dispensing and administering drugs beyond licence should select those drugs that offer the best balance of benefit against harm for any given patient
- Health professionals should inform, change and monitor their practice with regard to drugs used beyond licence in the light of evidence from audit and published research
- Organizations providing pain management services should support therapeutic practices that are underpinned by evidence and advocated by a responsible body of professional opinion

ASPIRATION, ACCURACY AND MISCELLANEOUS INJECTIONS

ASPIRATION

If a joint effusion is present then aspiration is useful both diagnostically and therapeutically[72]. An effusion in a joint is known to result in loss of muscle strength (arthrogenic muscle inhibition), so physiotherapy is unlikely to be successful unless any effusion is suppressed[118,119]. In OA of the knee there is controversy as to whether the presence of an effusion predicts a better response to joint injection than if the knee is dry[37,277]. In inflammatory arthritis the effect of an injection may be prolonged by 24 hours' bed rest immediately after the procedure, but the benefit of this in OA is less certain[278–280]. In RA of the knee, aspiration of synovial fluid prior to steroid injection significantly reduces the risk of relapse[120].

Joint fluid can be loculated, very viscous and contain debris, all of which can prevent complete aspiration. It might be impossible to aspirate anything with a small-bore needle, so use at least a 21-G or even a 19-G needle. Moving the tip of the needle a few millimetres, or rotating it through 90 degrees, can improve the flow into the syringe.

We recommend that disposable gloves are worn (to protect the clinician)[116], and that towels are used to protect the treatment area.

A three-way connector between needle and syringe is useful to avoid having to disconnect the syringe if it is full but there is still further fluid to aspirate. If this happens, the joint fluid tends to drip out of the disconnected needle (hence the need for something to catch the drips), so have another syringe ready to connect immediately. If the needle is left in the joint and the syringe is disconnected, the pressure between the inside and outside of the joint will equalize, and this might be why it is more difficult to aspirate.

After aspiration, immediately examine the fluid for *colour*, *clarity* and *viscosity*.

The clinical context will usually accurately predict the nature of the aspirate. The requirement for all aspirates is to be sent for microscopy and culture to exclude crystal arthritis[121] and infection has been challenged[215]. An estimated third of rheumatologists routinely send aspirated synovial fluid samples for culture irrespective of the underlying diagnosis. This is done even when sepsis is not suspected. An audit of 507 synovial fluid culture requests revealed that positive bacterial growth was rare even when sepsis was queried on the request forms, but none was positive in any of the routine samples, throwing doubt on the value of routine synovial fluid culture. One recommended policy is that such cultures are undertaken when infection is a possibility and in immunocompromised patients. It is estimated that an average health district would save £3000 per annum if such a policy was adopted, so across the UK as a whole the total expenditure saved on this investigation would be considerable[215]. Clinicians need to develop local policies in consultation with their colleagues.

Ideally, any aspirate should be examined in the laboratory within 4 hours of aspiration. If analysis is delayed there will be a decrease in cell count, crystal dissolution, and artefacts will start to appear. Storage at 4°C will delay but not prevent these changes. To exclude tuberculosis (TB), specifically request Ziehl–Nielsen (Z-N) staining and await prolonged – usually 6 weeks – culture (TB is more common in immunosuppressed patients, recent immigrants, people of Asian ancestry and alcoholics).

Synovial fluid analysis is of major diagnostic value in acute arthritis, where septic arthritis or crystal arthropathy is suspected[159]. Although many laboratory tests can be performed on synovial fluid, only the white blood cell count (and percentage of polymorphonuclear lymphocytes), presence or absence of crystals, Gram stain and bacterial culture are helpful (special cultures are needed if TB or fungal infection are suspected)[122,159]. A critical appraisal of the relevant literature concluded that given the importance of synovial fluid tests, rationalization of their use, together with improved quality control, should be immediate priorities. Further investigation was recommended into the contribution of synovial fluid inspection and white cell counts to diagnosis, as well as of the specificity and sensitivity of synovial fluid microbiological assays, crystal identification, and cytology[159].

The percentage of polymorph leucocytes in synovial fluid aspirated from rheumatoid knees might have a modest predictive value for the medium-term effectiveness of subsequent intra-articular steroid injection[191].

Inoculation of the aspirate from joints and bursae into liquid media bottles (blood culture bottles) increases the sensitivity in the detection of sepsis[123,124]. *Staphylococcus aureus* is the most common organism in cases of septic arthritis and monosodium urate monohydrate crystals are present in gout.

In small joints, such as in the hand, ultrasound guidance can improve the accuracy and frequency of joint aspiration[270,271].

WHAT THE ASPIRATE MIGHT BE

- *Serous fluid of variable viscosity*: normal or non-inflammatory synovial fluid is colourless or pale yellow (straw-coloured fluid). It contains few cells (less than 500/l, mainly mononuclear) and little debris and therefore appears clear. It does not clot and is very viscous due to its high hyaluronic acid content. The 'drip test' forms a string 2–5 cm long before separating. Should you aspirate and inject at the same time, or await the result of joint fluid analysis? This depends on the clinical context, appearance of the fluid and experience of the clinician. If in doubt, *do not* inject

- *Serous fluid streaked with fresh blood*: this is not uncommon and is usually related to the trauma of the aspiration. It can occur at the end of the procedure when the tap becomes dry, or during the procedure if the needle tip is moved

- *Frank blood*: there is usually a history of recent trauma with the joint swelling up within hours. Aspiration gives pain relief, allows joint movement and removes an irritant that causes synovitis. Blood often means a significant traumatic lesion so X-ray is mandatory. Haemarthrosis of the knee is due to anterior cruciate ligament rupture in 40% of cases. If there is a lipid layer on top of the blood this suggests intra-articular fracture. It is suggested that steroid injection following aspiration of a haemarthrosis might prevent a subsequent chemical synovitis and accelerate recovery[39]. Recommended practice might change if and when more evidence becomes available. Further management depends on the cause of the haemarthrosis. Rarely, haemarthrosis might be due to a bleeding disorder, anticoagulant treatment or from a vascular lesion in the joint, e.g. haemangioma

- *Xanthochromic fluid*: this is old blood that has broken down and appears orange in colour. Its presence implies old trauma

- *Turbid fluid*: inflammatory fluid tends to be less viscous than normal joint fluid, so it forms drops in the 'drip test'. It also looks darker and more turbid due to the increase in debris, cells and fibrin, and clots might form. It is impossible to say from the gross appearance what the inflammatory process is, so *do not* inject but await results of direct microscopy and culture studies

- *Frank pus*: rare in practice – the patient is likely to be very ill and needs urgent admission. The aspirate has a foul smell

- *Other*: uniformly milky-white fluid might result from plentiful cholesterol or urate crystals. Rice bodies are small, shiny, white objects composed of sloughed microinfarcted synovial villi. Greatly increased viscosity may be due to a recent steroid injection into that joint (or hypothyroidism)

UNEXPECTED ASPIRATION

Sometimes unexpected fluid might be aspirated, which then contaminates the injection solution. Using gloves and towels, the loaded syringe carefully disconnected should be from the needle, taking care not to displace the needle and desterilize the tip of the syringe. A fresh, empty 10–20-ml syringe is then locked tightly onto the needle without displacement, and aspiration made.

If the aspirate is 'suspect' do not inject. If it remains appropriate to inject, the original solution can be used, providing it is not too heavily contaminated and that the end of the syringe is kept sterile by attaching it to a sterile needle. If in doubt, a fresh solution should be drawn up and the syringe locked tightly onto the needle.

Very rarely, a blood vessel might be punctured, e.g. an artery at the wrist in a carpal tunnel injection. Fresh, bright red arterial blood will pump into the syringe, which should be withdrawn and firm pressure applied over the puncture site for several minutes.

ASPIRATING GANGLIA

Ganglion cysts account for approximately 60% of soft tissue, tumour-like swellings affecting the hand and wrist. They usually develop spontaneously in adults 20 to 50 years of age with a female:male preponderance of 3:1. The dorsal wrist ganglion arises from the scapholunate joint and constitutes about 65% of ganglia of the wrist and hand. The volar wrist ganglion arises from the distal aspect of the radius and accounts for about 20 to 25% of ganglia; flexor tendon sheath ganglia make up the remaining 10 to 15%. The cystic structures are found near or are attached to tendon sheaths and joint capsules. The cyst is filled with soft, gelatinous, sticky, and mucoid fluid[235].

Most ganglia resolve spontaneously and do not require treatment. If the patient has symptoms, including pain or paraesthesia, or is disturbed by the appearance, aspiration without injection of a corticosteroid might be effective[235]. In a study comparing aspiration of wrist ganglia with aspiration plus steroid injection, both treatments had a 33% success rate. Almost all ganglia that recurred after one aspiration did not resolve with further aspirations. After aspiration and explanation of the benign nature of ganglia, only 25% of patients requested surgery[125].

ACCURACY OF INJECTION

Relatively few studies have reported on the accuracy of joint and soft-tissue injection techniques and the relationship of injection accuracy to clinical outcomes. Interestingly, the experience and seniority of the injector does not appear to influence the accuracy of injection placement[12], and for most disorders the optimum injection technique has yet to be firmly established. The approaches described in this book are based on the extensive clinical experience of the authors, and on techniques described in the medical literature.

For the majority of joint injections it is sufficient to follow an anatomical landmark[297]. Even the hip, a joint considered relatively inaccessible without imaging[297], can be successfully injected 80% of the time using anatomical landmarks[298].

It is important to use a needle that is long enough, especially in obese patients, or the joint cavity might not be reached, e.g. in the knee a 2 inch (5-cm) needle might be required rather than a standard 1.5-inch (3.8-cm) needle[299].

Needle placement can be confirmed when an effusion is present. During joint aspiration, the appearance of synovial fluid indicates intra-articular placement of the needle[299]. Remarkably, however, even the ability to aspirate fluid is not a perfect predictor of intra-articular placement of a subsequent injection[12]. In the absence of an effusion, needle placement requires the use of anatomical landmarks and tactile feedback to help the clinician position the needle[299]. Minimal retraction of the needle after 'caressing' articular cartilage or bone with the needle tip may help to ensure intra-articular placement[299].

The choice of entry portal and positioning of a joint can affect accurate injection placement. In one study, injecting a dry knee in the extended position using a lateral midpatellar approach into the patellofemoral joint was intra-articular >90% of the time and more accurate than injecting through the 'eyes' of the knee (anteromedial and anterolateral to the patellar tendon) with the knee in partial flexion[299].

Accuracy of intra-articular knee injection can be confirmed by adding 1–2 ml of air to the injection. Immediately after injection a 'squishing' sound is audible from the knee when it is put through its range of motion. In one small study this simple test had a sensitivity of 85% and a specificity of 100%[147]. A similar test has been described in the shoulder[95]. The 'whoosh' test can be used to confirm accurate needle placement in caudal epidurals. This involves listening for a 'whoosh' with a stethoscope placed over the sacrum while a small amount of air is injected before the attempt to inject into the epidural space. In a small study of patients undergoing caudal epidural injection, 19 had correct needle placement as determined by epidurography. All of these had a positive 'whoosh' test and there were no false positives[306].

In some instances, an injection that is outside but close to the target may be effective. A good therapeutic response might be experienced when an attempted joint or tendon sheath injection has been periarticular or peri-tendinous, suggesting that total accuracy of needle placement might not be essential to a satisfactory outcome[12,300,301]. In some studies, however, better outcomes have been associated with more accurate injections[13,302].

When injecting hyalgans, the small amount of viscous fluid and the resistance to its flow in the needle can make it difficult to feel if the solution is passing into periarticular tissue or joint space. Incorrect placement can cause more discomfort during and after the procedure. It is thought that painful injections are associated with extra-articular needle placement and might be linked to a higher incidence of adverse reactions. Once the instantaneous discomfort of needle placement has subsided, the injection of hyalgans should not be painful[299].

A variety of imaging methods, including X-ray screening, computed tomography (CT) scanning and, more recently, ultrasound and magnetic resonance imaging (MRI), have been used to better localize needle placement. The question arises as to whether guided injection produces a significantly different result from those using anatomical landmarks[297]. There have been a few prospective randomized controlled trials to investigate this issue. In one, patients who were randomized to receive ultrasound-guided subacromial injection of steroid experienced greater improvement in shoulder function and pain than those who received a 'blind' injection[303]. In contrast, ultrasound-guided steroid injections for recalcitrant plantar fasciitis were no more effective than palpation-guided injections[16,304]. Similarly, CT guidance did not confer any added benefit over the anatomical landmark approach to suprascapular nerve block injection for chronic shoulder pain[305].

Image guidance can be useful when training clinicians to inject, in very obese patients, and to verify correct placement in research studies[15]. Ultrasound can be particularly helpful to monitor the effect of injection therapy[307-311]. However, until we have good evidence that imaging-guided injections in routine therapeutic practice are more effective both clinically and in cost terms, it seems reasonable to conclude that most injections should be given using an anatomical landmark approach; imaging-guided injection should be reserved for those patients who have not responded to this approach[297,303]. Further studies are needed to verify reproducible and accurate methods of therapeutic delivery into joint and soft-tissue lesions without the need for imaging confirmation.

Finally, it is important to recognize that patients' expectations and preferences can affect the outcome of injection therapy[312].

MISCELLANEOUS INJECTIONS

GOUT Joint aspiration in acute gout can ease pain and facilitate diagnosis. Aspiration of joints in the intercritical period (the interval between acute attacks) can also help make the diagnosis of gout. Intra-articular injection of steroid is an effective treatment; a single dose of triamcinolone acetonide 40 mg can resolve symptoms within 48 hours. Smaller doses, e.g. 10 mg in knee joints or 8 mg in smaller joints, can also be effective. Intra-articular injection requires precise diagnosis and should not be used if there is a suspicion of joint infection; the two can coexist[195,282].

MUCOID CYSTS Mucoid cysts are small swellings typically found on the distal interphalangeal joints of patients with OA. They are a form of ganglion and communicate directly with the joint. On the affected finger they are often associated with nail ridging or deformity, which frequently resolves after successful injection treatment. In one study, 60% had not recurred 2 years after receiving multiple punctures with a 25-G needle and a small volume (<1 ml) injection of steroid and local anaesthetic[284].

RHEUMATOID NODULES In one small study, superficial rheumatoid nodules injected with steroid and local anaesthetic significantly reduced in volume or disappeared, compared with nodules injected with placebo, and with no significant complications[212].

TRIGGER POINTS Trigger points are discrete, focal, hyper-irritable areas located in a taut band of skeletal muscle. They produce pain locally and in a referred pattern, and often accompany chronic musculoskeletal disorders. Trigger points can manifest as regional persistent pain, tension headache, tinnitus, temporomandibular joint pain, decreased range of motion in the legs and low back pain. Palpation of a hypersensitive bundle or nodule of muscle of harder than normal consistency is typical and can elicit pain locally and/or cause radiation of pain towards a zone of reference and a local twitch response. The commonly encountered locations of trigger points and their pain reference zones are consistent[286].

Injection of 1% lidocaine without steroid appears to be effective[287]. The trigger point is fixed by pinching it between the thumb and index finger; the needle is then inserted 1 to 2 cm away from the trigger point and advanced into the trigger point at an angle of 30° to the skin. Warn the patient of the possibility of sharp pain, muscle twitching or an unpleasant sensation as the needle contacts the taut muscular band. A small amount (0.2 ml) of local anaesthetic is injected when the needle is inside the trigger point. The needle is then withdrawn to the level of the subcutaneous tissue and redirected superiorly, inferiorly, laterally and medially, repeating the needling and injection process in each direction until the local twitch response is no longer elicited or resisting muscle tautness is no longer perceived. Repeated injections are not recommended if two or three previous attempts have been unsuccessful. Patients are encouraged to remain active, putting muscles through their full range of motion in the week following trigger-point injections[287].

INJECTION TECHNIQUE GUIDELINES

The following guidelines should be studied carefully before using any of the injection techniques.

To make the practical section of this book easy to use we have simplified each technique and presented only the essential facts. There now follows an explanation of each section, outlining the rationale behind this approach to injection therapy. Each page covers one anatomical structure with the most common lesion found there.

Please note that *none* of the doses, volumes, equipment and general advice is 'cast in stone'. Amounts injected depend on the size, age and general health of the patient, and are based on the patients we commonly inject in orthopaedic medicine outpatient settings. With experience, the clinician will be able to adapt ways of using the methods shown.

At the beginning of upper and lower limb and spinal sections, a brief outline of the assessment procedure and list of capsular patterns for each joint is listed.

The *capsular pattern* is a set pattern of limitation of range for each individual joint, which occurs when this joint suffers from capsulitis. The cause of the capsulitis could be OA, systemic arthritis or trauma, but the ratio of limitation in the joint remains the same.

CAUSES AND FINDINGS

Giving injections is easy; it is the *selection* of the appropriate patient that is difficult; therefore great care must be used in the assessment.

This section lists the common causes of the lesion and the main findings of the assessment to aid clinicians in this patient selection. After the examination, the different treatment options should be discussed, contraindications to injection eliminated, possible complications and outcomes detailed and the patient's consent to an injection gained (see the Contraindications section, p 38).

EQUIPMENT

Tables 10 and 11 show the recommended size of syringe and needle, dosage and volume of corticosteroid and local anaesthetic, and total volume. These doses and volumes are usual for the average-sized adult and should be adapted for smaller or larger frames.

First, decide on the volume (how large is the structure to be injected?) and then the appropriate dose (how many milligrams of the drug are suitable, using the minimal effective dose?). Then choose a syringe of a size appropriate for the volume to be injected and a needle of the correct length to reach the structure. All needles and syringes must be of single-use disposable type and must be checked to ensure they are in date.

SYRINGES Have available 1-ml, 2-ml, 5-ml, 10-ml and 20-ml syringes; occasionally a 50-ml syringe might be necessary for aspiration.

Use a small-bore, 1-ml tuberculin syringe for small tendons and ligaments because the resistance of the structure can require a certain amount of pressure. Considerable back pressure can cause a larger-bore syringe to blow off the needle, and thus the clinician and patient to be sprayed with the solution – an embarrassing situation.

NEEDLES Select the finest needle of the appropriate length to reach the lesion (Table 10). Even on a slim person, it is often necessary to use a 3.5-inch (90-mm) or longer needle to successfully infiltrate deep structures such as the hip joint or psoas bursa. It is better to use a longer needle than might appear necessary, than one that is too short, which could necessitate withdrawing and starting again. When injecting with a long, fine, spinal needle it might be useful to keep the trochar in place to help control the needle as it passes through tissue planes.

	Colour	Gauge	Width	Length
Table 10 Needle sizes and colours most commonly used and available in the UK (Note: other countries may use different hub colours)	Orange	25G	0.5 mm	0.5 to {5/8} inch (13–20 mm)
	Blue	23G	0.6 mm	1 to 1.25 inches (25–30 mm)
	Green	21G	0.8 mm	1.5 to 2 inches (39–50 mm)
	White	19G	1.1 mm	1.5 inches (40 mm)
	Black	Spinal 21 or 22G	0.7–0.8 mm	3–4 inches (75–100 mm)

CORTICOSTEROID We suggest the use of Kenalog 40 (triamcinolone acetonide with 40 mg per ml) throughout the technique sections.

Any appropriate corticosteroid can be used but, in our experience, Kenalog gives less postinjection flare in soft-tissue injections, especially into soft tissues, than Depo-Medrone and is equally effective. Another advantage is that Kenalog can be used in both small *and* large areas. Adcortyl (triamcinolone acetonide with 10 mg steroid per ml) can be used where the total volume to be injected is over 5 ml; this allows greater volume for the same dose and avoids the need to dilute the local anaesthetic with normal saline.

LOCAL ANAESTHETIC

We suggest the use of lidocaine hydrochloride (without epinephrine) through-out, but any suitable local anaesthetic can be used. We recommend the following maximum doses:

- 2% lidocaine up to a maximum volume of 2 ml
- 1% lidocaine for 2- to 5-ml maximum volumes
- dilute 1% with normal saline (0.9%) for volumes larger than 5 ml or use Adcortyl

These recommended maximum doses are less than half those published in pharmacological texts[91], so are well within safety limits. Occasionally Marcain can be used when a longer anaesthetic effect is needed but, because of its longer half-life, we do not normally use it for these injections. Some practitioners like to mix short- and long-acting anaesthetics to gain both the immediate diagnostic effect and the longer therapeutic effect.

In a study using large volumes of local anaesthetic during knee surgery, patients were injected with 45 ml of 1% lidocaine (with epinephrine) plus 45 ml of 0.25 bupivacaine (50 ml of the total volume into the joint and 40 ml into the soft tissues around the knee). Over the 2 hours following injection, serial measurements of serum levels of the anaesthetic agents in all patients at all time intervals were well within the ranges considered safe[160].

Where any doubt exists about the possibility of the patient being allergic to local anaesthetic, *do not use it*. Volume can be obtained with normal saline if necessary.

DOSAGE AND VOLUME

The doses and volumes given in this section are intended for the average-sized adult and should be viewed as guidelines only. They are governed by the size, age and general health of the patient, the number of injections to be given and by clinical judgement. At all times, the *minimum* effective dose should be given; this will help prevent the appearance of adverse side effects such as facial flushing, intermenstrual bleeding and hyperglycaemia.

Tendons and ligaments should have small amounts of local anaesthetic and steroid injected. A small volume avoids painful distension of the structure and a small dose minimizes risk of rupture. An average 'recipe' for most tendon lesions is 10 mg of steroid in a total of 1 ml of local anaesthetic. Larger structures might require up to 20 mg of steroid in 2 ml volume.

Joints and bursae appear to respond best when sufficient fluid to bathe the inflamed internal surfaces is introduced. Possibly the slight distension 'splints' the structure, or breaks down or stretches out adhesions.

Recommended average dosages and volumes for joint injections are shown in Table 11. In a small patient the amounts are decreased and in a large patient they may be increased. These volumes are well within safety limits and will not cause the capsule to rupture; for instance it is not unusual to aspirate over 100 ml of blood from an injured knee joint. In any case, the back pressure created by too large a volume would blow the syringe off the fine needle recommended, long before the capsule was compromised.

Joint	Dosage	Volume
Shoulder	40 mg	5 ml
Elbow	30 mg	4 ml
Wrist	20 mg	2 ml
Thumb	10 mg	1 ml
Fingers	5 mg	0.5 ml
Hip	40 mg	5 ml
Knee	40 mg	10 ml
Ankle	30 mg	4 ml
Foot	20 mg	2 ml
Toes	10 mg	1 ml

Table 11 Recommended average dosages and volumes for joint injections

ANATOMY

As an aid to identifying the structures, we give tips for ways to imagine these individual sizes and to localize them, based on functional and surface anatomy. Where finger sizes are given, they refer to the patient's fingers, not the clinician's.

TECHNIQUE

This section describes, in a logical sequence, the procedure for administration of the solution. The steps are presented as bullet points for ease of execution.

Injections should not be painful. Skin is very sensitive, especially on the flexor surfaces of the body, and bone is equally so. Muscles, tendons and ligaments are less sensitive and cartilage virtually insensitive. Pain caused at the time of the injection is invariably the result of poor technique – 'hitting' bone with the needle instead of 'caressing' it. Afterpain can be caused by a traumatic periostitis because of damaging bone with the needle, or possibly by flare caused by the type of steroid used. Success does not depend on a painful flare after the infiltration, although some patients do experience this. It is good practice to warn patients of possible afterpain and to ensure that they have painkillers available should they need them.

The secret of giving a reasonably comfortable injection depends on using the needle as an extension of the finger. The needle should be inserted *rapidly* and *perpendicular* to strongly *stretched skin*, and then passed gently through the tissue planes, feeding back information about the structures from the consistency of those tissues. The usual 'feel' of different tissues is as follows:

- muscle: spongy, soft
- tendon or ligament: fibrous, tough
- capsule: sometimes slight resistance to needle, like pushing through the skin of a balloon
- cartilage: sticky, toffee-like
- bone: hard and extremely sensitive

Bursae and *joint capsules* are hollow structures that require the solution to be deposited in one amount – a *bolus technique*. No resistance to the introduction of fluid indicates that the needle tip is within a space. Chronic bursitis, especially at the shoulder, can result in loculation of the bursa. This gives the sensation of pockets of free flow and then resistance within the bursa, rather like injecting a sponge.

Tendons and *ligaments* require a *peppering technique*. This helps to disperse the solution throughout the structure and to eliminate the possibility of rupture. The needle is gently inserted to caress the bone at the enthesis and the solution is then introduced in little droplets, as if into all parts of a cube (see Figure 1). Knowing the three-dimensional size of the structure is essential as this indicates the volume of fluid required and how much the needle tip has to be moved around. There is only one skin puncture; this is not multiple acupuncture.

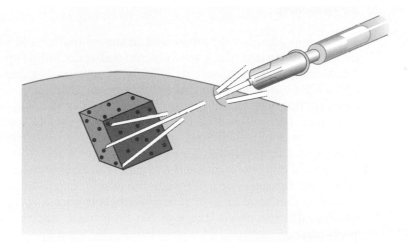

Tendons with sheaths: after inserting the needle perpendicular to the skin, lay the needle alongside the tendon within the sheath and introduce the fluid. Often a small bulge is observed contained within the sheath.

Blood vessels: avoid puncturing a large blood vessel – if this occurs, apply firm pressure over the site for 5 min (vein) or 10 min (artery).

Aspiration: check any aspirated fluid – if sepsis is suspected, aspirate with a fresh syringe and deposit in a sterile container for culture. Abandon the injection (see Aspiration section).

MAXIMIZING PATIENT COMFORT DURING AN INJECTION

Maintain a calm confident approach throughout the procedure and follow these three rules:

● strongly stretch skin between finger and thumb
● hold needle perpendicular to skin
● insert needle rapidly

The needle can then be turned towards the lesion and gently and slowly advanced through the tissue planes.

Asking the patient to cough just as the needle is inserted has been shown to make venesection less painful, possibly through a combination of distraction and raising intraspinal pressure to momentarily block pain transmission[171]; it might also make injection therapy less painful. Emla local anaesthetic cream can be used for sensitive sites such as the hand, and might be helpful for patients who are especially apprehensive; it must be applied at least 1 hour before the procedure under occlusion[205]. Playing classical music during an injection clinic has proved to be unsuccessful[207].

Spraying the injection site with ethyl chloride rapidly cools it and has been used for many years to make injections less painful, although it has not been systematically studied in injection therapy. Anaesthetizing the skin and subcutaneous tissues with local anaesthetic before knee aspiration does not make the procedure less painful[283].

AFTERCARE

This section addresses the advice and treatment that should be given to the patient after the injection is administered and at the follow-up appointment. Injections give demonstrable relief in the short term but there is not much difference from other treatments or no treatment at all in the long term. It is essential, therefore, to address the cause or causes of the pain once the symptoms have been relieved by the injection. Recurrence of symptoms is very common in certain conditions, such as bursitis and tendinopathy, so appropriate advice on prevention is part of the care package.

The ideal outcome is total relief of pain with normal power and full range of motion. This does not always occur but when local anaesthetic is used there should be significant immediate improvement to encourage both patient and clinician that the correct diagnosis has been made, and the injection accurately placed.

Explain the probable after effects of the injection to the patient. The relief of pain might be temporary, depending on the strength and type of anaesthetic used, and the pain might return when this effect wears off. Some patients describe this pain as greater than their original pain; this might be due to the flare effect, which is thought to be caused by microcrystal deposition. It is also possible that pain that comes back after some relief might *appear* to be worse. Any afterpain is usually transient and can be eased by application of ice or taking simple analgesia.

The anti-inflammatory effect of the corticosteroid is not usually apparent until 24–48 h after the infiltration and will continue for 3 weeks to 3 months, depending on the drug used.

Arrange to review the patient about 1 or 2 weeks later, or sooner if the pain is severe or begins to return – as in acute capsulitis of the shoulder.

Advise the patient on what to do and what to avoid. Joint conditions usually benefit from a programme of early *gentle movement* within the pain-free range; studies have shown that 24-hours' complete bed rest after a knee injection for inflammatory arthritis is beneficial[278-281] but in the case of the wrist immobilization does not appear to improve outcome and might even worsen it[162]. Overuse conditions in tendons and bursae require *relative rest*; this means that normal activities of daily living can be followed, provided they are not too painful. The patient should be encouraged to do anything that is comfortable.

When the symptoms have been relieved, the patient will usually need a few sessions of treatment for rehabilitation and prevention of recurrence; this is particularly relevant in overuse conditions and might involve correction of posture, ergonomic advice, adaptation of movement patterns, mobilization or manipulation, deep friction massage, stretching and/or strengthening regimes. The advice of a professional coach in their chosen sport or an expert in orthotics might also be required. Sporting or repetitive activities should not be engaged upon until the patient is symptom-free.

COMMENTS

This section describes the expected results of the treatment and any complications or difficulties that might occur.

ALTERNATIVE APPROACHES

Alternative ways of injecting the lesion or appropriate alternative approaches to treatment are described.

CONTRAINDICATIONS TO INJECTION THERAPY

ABSOLUTE CONTRAINDICATIONS

- Hypersensitivity to local anaesthetic: steroid alone can be used
- Sepsis: local or systemic (do not inject patients with a suspected febrile illness, e.g. chest or urinary infection)
- Fracture site: can delay bone healing
- Prosthetic joint: risk of infection
- Children: injectable lesions that are not due to systemic arthropathy are exceedingly rare under the age of 18 years. Children spontaneously heal well; consider alternative diagnoses with blood tests and diagnostic imaging. Injection therapy for treatment of juvenile arthritis is not included in this book
- Reluctant patient: no informed consent given
- Gut feeling: when in doubt, do not inject

RELATIVE CONTRAINDICATIONS

- Diabetes: greater risk of sepsis, blood sugar levels may rise for a few days or, rarely, longer
- Immunosuppressed: by disease (leukaemia, AIDS) or by drugs (systemic steroids)
- Large tendinopathies: e.g. tendo-Achilles, infrapatella tendon (image first)
- Bleeding disorder: correct before injecting
- Anticoagulation therapy: but there is no good evidence of an increased bleeding risk
- Haemarthrosis: but this is disputed[39]; the pain relief obtained from aspiration can be dramatic. Fracture should be eliminated
- Psychogenic pain: injection can make the pain appear worse

PREPARATION PROTOCOL

PREPARE PATIENT
- Discuss various treatment options, injection procedure and possible side effects
- Obtain informed consent
- Place in comfortable sitting or lying position with injection site accessible

PREPARE EQUIPMENT
- Corticosteroid vials and single-use local anaesthetic ampoules
- Check names, doses and expiry dates
- In date syringe and needles for drawing up and infiltrating
- Alcohol swab or iodine skin preparation
- Cotton wool and skin plaster
- Spare syringe and sterile container for possible aspiration if appropriate

PREPARE SITE
- Identify structure and put skin under strong traction between finger and thumb
- Mark injection site with closed end of sterile needle cap, then discard
- Clean skin with suitable preparation in an outward spiral motion
- Allow skin one minute to dry

ASSEMBLE EQUIPMENT
- Wash hands with suitable cleanser for 1 min and dry well with disposable towel
- Open ampoule(s) and vial(s)
- Attach sterile 21-G green needle to appropriate-sized syringe
- Draw up accurate dose of steroid first, then discard vial
- Draw up accurate dose of local anaesthetic from single-use ampoule, then discard
- Attach fresh sterile needle of correct length firmly to syringe

INJECTION TECHNIQUE FLOWCHART

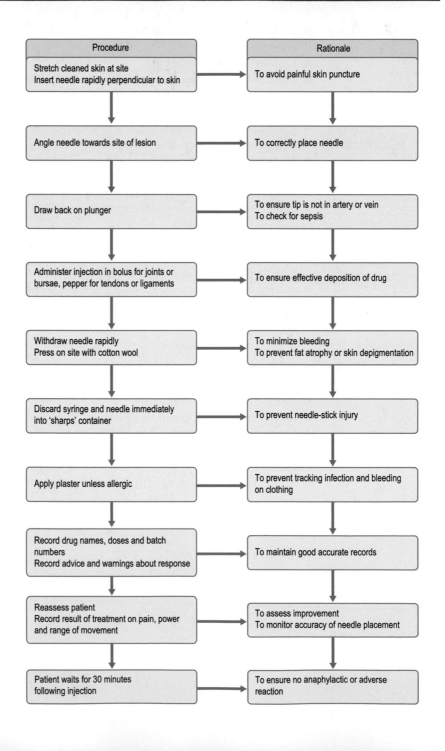

Procedure	Rationale
Stretch cleaned skin at site Insert needle rapidly perpendicular to skin	To avoid painful skin puncture
Angle needle towards site of lesion	To correctly place needle
Draw back on plunger	To ensure tip is not in artery or vein To check for sepsis
Administer injection in bolus for joints or bursae, pepper for tendons or ligaments	To ensure effective deposition of drug
Withdraw needle rapidly Press on site with cotton wool	To minimize bleeding To prevent fat atrophy or skin depigmentation
Discard syringe and needle immediately into 'sharps' container	To prevent needle-stick injury
Apply plaster unless allergic	To prevent tracking infection and bleeding on clothing
Record drug names, doses and batch numbers Record advice and warnings about response	To maintain good accurate records
Reassess patient Record result of treatment on pain, power and range of movement	To assess improvement To monitor accuracy of needle placement
Patient waits for 30 minutes following injection	To ensure no anaphylactic or adverse reaction

INJECTION TECHNIQUES OF THE UPPER LIMB

Finger measurements are from the patient, not the clinician.

ASSESSMENT OF THE UPPER LIMB

Shoulder tests

Active flexion above head
Passive flexion with overpressure
Active abduction to ear for painful arc
Passive lateral rotation
Passive abduction
Passive medial rotation

Resisted abduction
Resisted lateral rotation
Resisted medial rotation
Resisted elbow flexion
Resisted elbow extension
Resisted adduction

Shoulder capsular pattern: most loss of lateral rotation, less of abduction and least of medial rotation

Elbow tests

Passive flexion
Passive extension
Passive pronation
Passive supination

Resisted flexion
Resisted extension
Resisted pronation
Resisted supination
Resisted wrist flexion
Resisted wrist extension

Elbow capsular pattern: more loss of flexion than extension

Wrist tests

Passive pronation
Passive supination
Passive extension
Passive flexion
Passive radial deviation
Passive ulnar deviation

Resisted extension
Resisted flexion
Resisted radial deviation
Resisted ulnar deviation

Wrist capsular pattern: equal loss of flexion and extension

Digit tests

Passive thumb extension
Resisted thumb abduction
Resisted thumb adduction
Resisted thumb extension
Resisted thumb flexion

Passive finger extension
Passive finger flexion
Resisted finger abduction
Resisted finger adduction

Digit capsular pattern:
Loss of extension and abduction at thumb
Loss of *extension* and *radial deviation* at metacarpo-phalangeal joints
Loss of *flexion* at interphalangeal joints
Loss of *extension* at distal phalangeal joints

SECTION 2

GLENOHUMERAL JOINT

Acute or chronic capsulitis – 'frozen shoulder'

Causes and findings
- Trauma, osteoarthritis or rheumatoid arthritis
- Idiopathic or secondary to neurological disease, diabetes, stroke, etc
- Pain in deltoid area, possibly radiating down to hand in severe cases, aggravated by arm movements and lying on shoulder
- Painful limitation in the capsular pattern – most: loss of lateral rotation; less: loss of abduction; least: loss of medial rotation, with a hard end-feel

Equipment

Syringe	Needle	Kenalog 40	Lidocaine	Total volume
5 ml	21G 1.5–2 inches (40–50 mm) Green	40 mg	4 ml 1%	5 ml

Anatomy
The shoulder joint is surrounded by a large capsule and the easiest and least painful approach is posteriorly, where there are no major blood vessels or nerves. An imaginary oblique line running anteriorly from the posterior angle of the acromion to the coracoid process passes through the shoulder joint. The needle follows this line, passing through deltoid, infraspinatus and posterior capsule. The end point should be the sticky feel of cartilage on the head of the humerus or the glenoid.

Technique
- Patient sits with arms folded across waist, thus opening up the posterior joint space
- Identify posterior angle of acromion with thumb, and coracoid process with index finger
- Insert needle directly below angle and push obliquely anterior towards coracoid process until needle gently touches intra-articular cartilage
- Inject solution as a bolus

Aftercare
Patient maintains mobility with pendular and stretching exercises within the pain-free range, progressing to stronger stretching when pain is reduced. Strong passive stretching of the capsule can be given when the pain has abated. A strengthening and stabilizing programme is often required, together with postural correction.

Comments
The less the radiation of pain and the earlier the joint is treated, the more dramatic is the relief of symptoms. If there is resistance to the injection, the needle has probably been inserted too laterally and must be repositioned more medially. Occasionally there is slight resistance when the needle passes through the capsule. Usually one injection suffices in the early stages of the condition, but if necessary more can safely be given at increasing intervals of 1 week, 10 days, 2 weeks, etc.; it is sometimes necessary in advanced capsulitis to give four to six injections over about 2 months. Advise the patient that a repeat dose might be needed if the symptoms are severe and gradually return as the effect of the drug wears off.

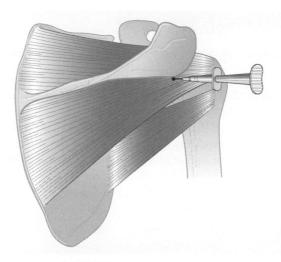

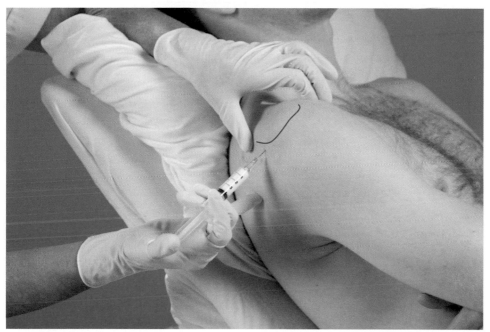

Alternative approaches   Rarely the posterior approach is not effective, so an anterior approach is used. In this case, the arm is held in slight lateral rotation and the needle inserted on the anterior surface between the coracoid process and the lesser tuberosity of the humerus, and aimed postero-medially towards the spine of the scapula. The same dose and volume is used. The disadvantages to this approach are that the patient can see the needle advancing, the flexor skin surfaces are more sensitive and there are more neuro-vascular structures lying on the anterior aspect of the shoulder.

Adcortyl (10 mg per ml) can be used for this injection, especially in large shoulders where more volume is required; the dose would then be 4 ml of Adcortyl with 4 ml of 1% local anaesthetic. Smaller patients may require only 30 mg of corticosteroid.

SECTION 2

SUPRASCAPULAR NERVE

Acute or chronic capsulitis of the glenohumeral joint

Causes and findings
- Trauma, osteoarthritis or rheumatoid arthritis
- Idiopathic or secondary to neurological disease, diabetes, stroke, etc. – 'frozen shoulder'
- Pain in deltoid area possibly radiating down to hand in severe cases
- Painful limitation in the capsular pattern – most: loss of lateral rotation; less: loss of abduction; least: loss of medial rotation, with a hard end-feel

Equipment

Syringe	Needle	Kenalog 40	Lidocaine	Total volume
1 ml	21G 1.75 inches (40 mm) Green	20 mg	Nil	0.5 ml

Anatomy
The suprascapular nerve passes through the suprascapular notch into the supraspinous fossa, runs laterally to curl around the neck of the spine of the scapula and ends in the infraspinous fossa. It supplies the supraspinatus and infraspinatus, and sends articular branches to the shoulder and acromioclavicular joints. It is worth injecting here when intracapsular injections have not been successful.

Technique
- The patient sits supported with arm in neutral position
- Identify lateral end of spine of scapular, move one-third along medially and mark a spot one finger superiorly in suprascapular fossa
- Insert needle perpendicular to fossa and touch bone
- Inject solution as a bolus

Aftercare
Mobility at the shoulder is maintained within pain-free range. Stretching and mobilization are started when pain permits.

Comments
Symptoms of paraesthesia or burning when inserting the needle indicate that it is within the nerve. Withdraw slightly before injecting.

A small randomized trial suggests that suprascapular nerve block is a safe and effective alternative treatment for frozen shoulder in primary care[126]. Some clinicians advise the use of a longer-lasting anaesthetic alone or with corticosteroid. This injection might also be useful in patients with rotator cuff tears who are not fit for surgery.

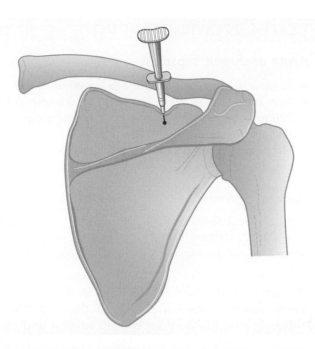

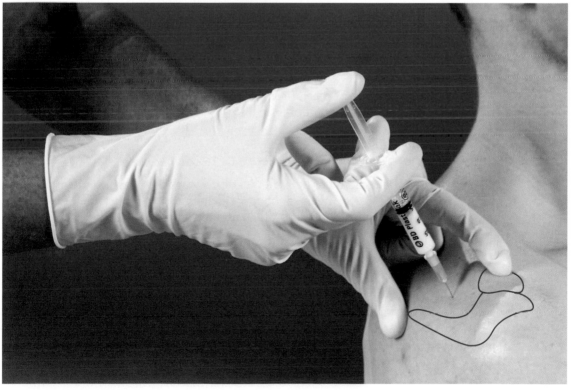

ACROMIOCLAVICULAR JOINT

Acute or chronic capsulitis

Causes and findings
- Trauma or occasionally prolonged overuse in a degenerative shoulder
- Pain at point of shoulder: occasionally a bump of bone or swelling is seen
- Painful: end-range of all passive movements, especially full passive horizontal adduction (scarf test)
- Occasionally painful: arc on active elevation especially towards end of range

Equipment

Syringe	Needle	Kenalog 40	Lidocaine	Total volume
1 ml	25G 0.5 inch (16mm) Orange	10mg	0.75ml 2%	1 ml

Anatomy
The acromioclavicular joint line runs in the sagittal plane about a thumb's width medial to the lateral edge of the acromion. The joint plane runs obliquely medially from superior to inferior and usually contains a small meniscus. Often a small step can be palpated where the acromion abuts against the clavicle, or a small V-shaped gap felt at the anterior joint margin. Passively gliding the acromion downwards on the clavicle may help in finding the joint line.

Technique
- Patient sits supported with arm hanging by side to slightly separate the joint surfaces
- Identify lateral edge of acromion. Move medially about a thumb's width and mark mid-point of joint line
- Insert needle angling medially about 30° from the vertical and pass through capsule
- Inject solution as a bolus

Aftercare
The patient should rest the shoulder for a week then begin gentle mobilizing exercises. Acutely inflamed joints are helped by the application of ice, taping to stabilize the joint and by oral pain killers.

Comments
Occasionally the joint is difficult to enter; it is normally a narrow space and degenerative changes make it more so. Traction on the arm can open up the joint space and peppering of the capsule with the solution will anaesthetize it while feeling for the joint space with the needle. This will avoid giving unnecessary pain.

Alternative approach
The joint can also be injected anteriorly and horizontally at the V-shaped gap if the superior approach is difficult. The unstable or repeatedly subluxing joint can be helped by sclerosing injections or possibly surgery.

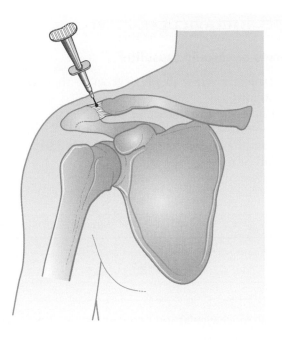

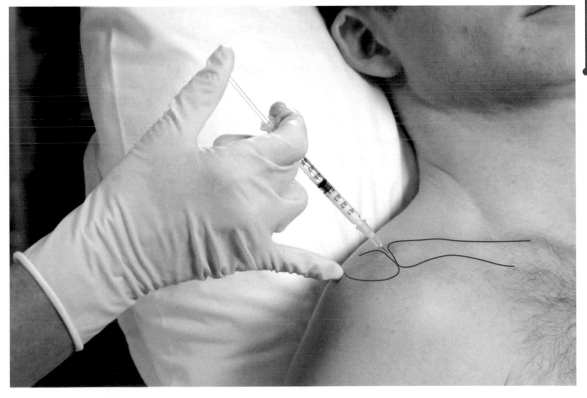

STERNOCLAVICULAR JOINT

Acute or chronic capsulitis

Causes and findings
- Trauma, overuse in the degenerate shoulder or occasionally rheumatoid arthritis
- Pain over sternoclavicular joint
- Painful:
  retraction and protraction of the shoulder
  full elevation of the arm
  clicking or subluxation after trauma

Equipment

Syringe	Needle	Kenalog 40	Lidocaine	Total volume
1 ml	25G 0.5 inch (16 mm) Orange	10 mg	0.5 ml 2%	0.75 ml

Anatomy The sternoclavicular joint contains a small meniscus that can sometimes be damaged and then give painful symptoms. The joint line runs obliquely laterally from superior to inferior and can be identified by palpating the joint medial to the end of the clavicle while the patient protracts and retracts the shoulder.

Technique
- Patient sits supported with arm in slight lateral rotation
- Identify mid-point of joint line
- Insert needle perpendicularly through joint capsule
- Inject solution as a bolus

Aftercare Rest for a week followed by mobilization and a progressive postural and exercise regime. Taping the joint helps stabilize it in the acute stage after trauma.

Comments Although not a common lesion, this usually responds well to one infiltration.

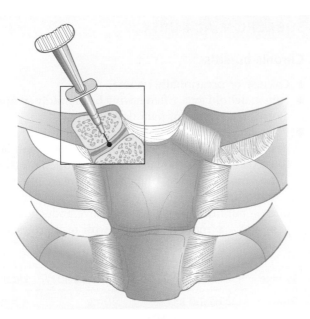

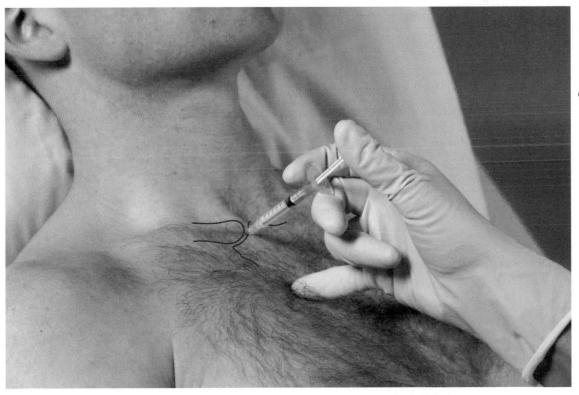

SUBACROMIAL BURSA

Chronic bursitis

Causes and findings
- Overuse or occasionally trauma
- Pain in deltoid area, often having been mildly symptomatic for a long time. Occasional referral of pain down arm
- Painful:
  passive elevation and medial rotation more than lateral rotation
  resisted abduction and lateral rotation, often on release of resistance. These two muscle groups often appear weak, but this is caused by muscle inhibition
  often – but not always – arc on active abduction
  generally – a 'muddle' of signs, with resisted tests repeated under distraction being less painful

Equipment

Syringe	Needle	Kenalog 40	Lidocaine	Total volume
5 ml	21G 1.5 inches (40 mm) Green	20 mg	4.5 ml 1%	5 ml

Anatomy The bursa lies mainly under the acromion but is very variable in size and can extend distally to the insertion of deltoid. Occasionally, a tender area can be palpated around the edge of the acromion. Sometimes the bursa communicates with the glenohumeral joint capsule.

Technique
- Patient sits with arm hanging by side to distract humerus from acromion
- Identify lateral edge of acromion
- Insert needle at mid-point of acromion and angle slightly upwards under acromion to full length
- Slowly withdraw needle while simultaneously injecting as a bolus wherever there is no resistance

Aftercare The patient must maintain retraction and depression of the shoulders and avoid elevation of the arm above shoulder level for up to 2 weeks. Taping the shoulder in retraction/depression for a few days, with postural advice, is helpful. When pain free, the patient commences resisted lateral rotation and retraction exercises, followed by strengthening of abduction. Retraining of overarm activities to avoid recurrence is essential.

Comments In our experience, this is the most common injectable lesion seen in orthopaedic medicine (see Appendix 1). Results are usually excellent; relief of pain after one injection is usual but the rehabilitation programme must be maintained. If, rarely, the symptoms persist after two injections, the shoulder should be scanned because a cuff tear might be present. In thin patients, the fluid sometimes causes visible swelling around the edge of the acromion.

Alternative approaches There is often loculation in long-standing bursitis. In this case, resistance is felt when injecting the solution, so the needle must be fanned around under the acromion to pepper separate pockets of the bursa – the sensation is that of injecting a sponge. Occasionally, calcification occurs within the bursa and hard resistance is felt. Infiltration with a large-bore needle and local anaesthetic may help. Failing this, surgical clearance is recommended. If palpable

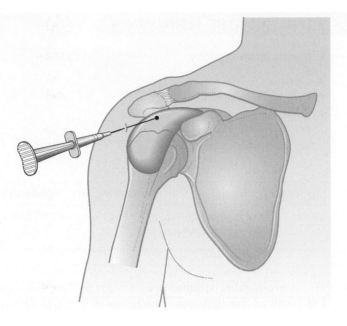

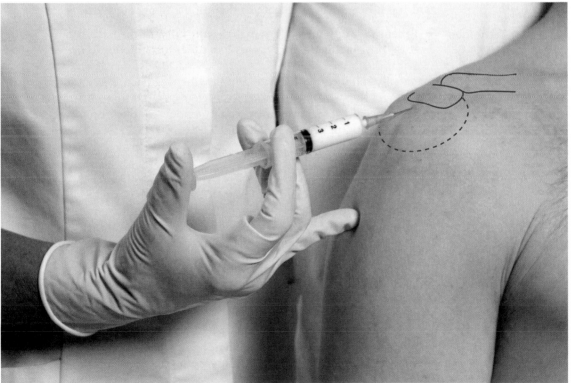

tenderness is found either anterior or posterior to the acromion, the injection can be given at these sites.

Acute subacromial bursitis is much less common and presents with spontaneous, rapidly increasing severe pain over a few days, which may radiate down as far as the wrist. The patient is often unable to move the arm at all and sleep is very disturbed. It should be injected in the same way as above but using a smaller total volume of 2 ml.

SUPRASPINATUS TENDON

Chronic tendinopathy

Cause and findings
- Overuse
- Pain in deltoid area
- Painful:
  resisted abduction
  arc on active abduction

Equipment

Syringe	Needle	Kenalog 40	Lidocaine	Total volume
1 ml	25G 0.5 inch (16mm) Orange	10mg	0.75ml 2%	1 ml

Anatomy
The supraspinatus tendon inserts into the superior facet on the greater tuberosity of the humerus, which lies in a direct line with the lateral epicondyle of the elbow. A line joining the two points passes through the tendon, which is approximately the size of the middle finger at insertion.

Technique
- Patient sits supported at about 45° with forearm medially rotated behind back, bringing the tendon forward so it lies just anterior to the edge of the acromion
- Identify rounded tendon in the hollow between acromion and tuberosity, in direct line with the lateral epicondyle
- Insert needle perpendicularly through tendon to touch bone
- Pepper solution perpendicularly into tendon

Aftercare
Relative rest is advised for up to 2 weeks. A progressive exercise and postural control regime is begun when symptom-free.

Comments
There is much controversy about injecting tendons because of the possibility of rupture. If the patient is elderly and the cause is traumatic, an ultrasound scan should be performed to determine if there is a tear in the tendon. Deep friction and a muscle balancing regime may then be the better treatment but surgery may be advised in some cases.

Alternative approaches
Supraspinatus tendinopathy can occur on its own but is often associated with subacromial bursitis. If there is doubt about the existence of a double lesion, the bursa should be injected first. If some pain remains on resisted abduction, then the tendon can be infiltrated a week or so later.

Calcification can arise within the tendon and a hard resistance would then be felt with the needle. It is worth attempting to break up the calcification with a large-bore needle and local anaesthetic. The results are variable. If symptoms persist a surgical opinion should be sought.

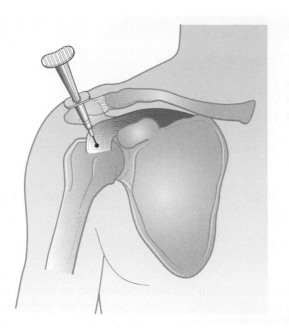

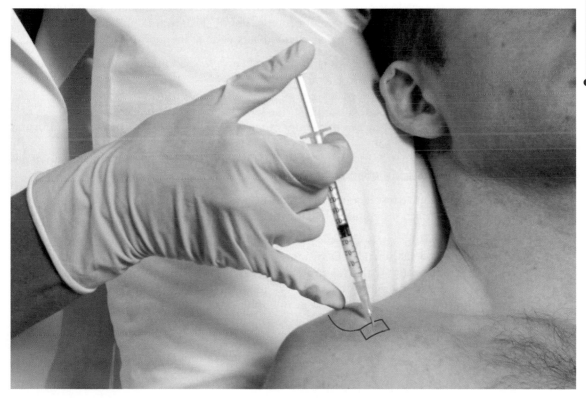

INFRASPINATUS TENDON

Chronic tendinopathy

Cause and findings
- Overuse
- Pain in deltoid area
- Painful:
  resisted lateral rotation
  arc on active abduction

Equipment

Syringe	Needle	Kenalog 40	Lidocaine	Total volume
2 ml	23G 1.25 inches (30 mm) Blue	20 mg	1.5 ml 2%	2 ml

Anatomy
The infraspinatus and teres minor tendons insert together into the middle and lower facets on the posterior aspect of the greater tuberosity of the humerus. Placing the arm in 90° of flexion, full adduction and lateral rotation brings the tendons out from under the thickest portion of the deltoid and puts them under tension. The tendons run obliquely upwards and laterally and are, together, approximately three fingers wide at the teno-osseous insertion.

Technique
- Patient sits or lies with supported arm flexed to right angle and held in full adduction and lateral rotation
- Identify posterior angle of acromion. Tendon insertion now lies 45° inferior and lateral in direct line with lateral epicondyle of the elbow
- Insert needle at mid-point of tendon at insertion. Pass through tendon and touch bone
- Pepper solution perpendicularly in two rows up and down into teno-osseous junction

Aftercare
Relative rest is advised for up to 2 weeks. A progressive exercise and postural correction regime is begun when symptom-free.

Alternative approaches
Usually a painful arc is present which indicates that the lesion lies at the teno-osseous junction. Occasionally there is no arc, when the lesion lies more in the body of the tendon. In this case, the needle is inserted more medially where there is often an area of tenderness. The same technique is applied.

This lesion might occur in conjunction with subacromial bursitis. If there is a possibility of a double lesion, inject the bursa first and the tendon later if symptoms persist.

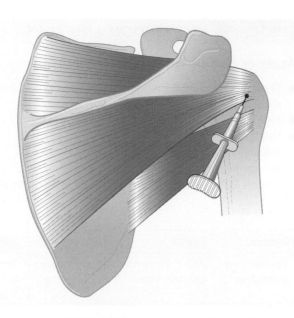

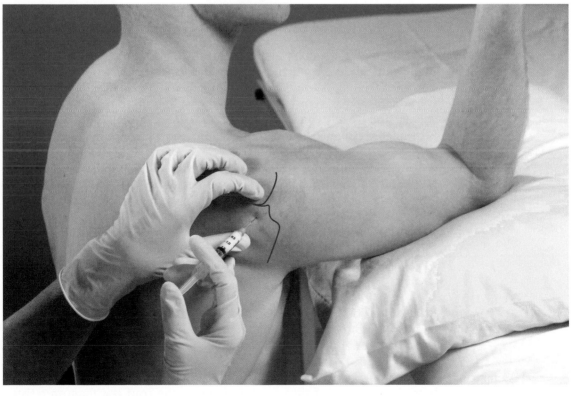

SUBSCAPULARIS TENDON AND BURSA

Acute or chronic tendinopathy or bursitis

Causes and findings
- Overuse or trauma: haemorrhagic bursitis can follow a direct blow to the shoulder
- Pain in deltoid area or anterior to shoulder
- Painful:
  resisted medial rotation
  arc on active abduction
  passive lateral rotation and full passive horizontal adduction (scarf test)

Equipment

Syringe	Needle	Kenalog 40	Lidocaine	Total volume
Tendon 1 ml Bursa 2 ml	23G 1.25 inches (30 mm) Blue	Tendon 10 mg Bursa 20 mg	Tendon 0.75 ml 2% Bursa 1.5 ml 2%	Tendon 1 ml Bursa 2 ml

Anatomy
The subscapularis tendon inserts into the medial edge of the lesser tuberosity of the humerus. It is approximately two fingers wide at its teno-osseous insertion and is a thin, fibrous structure feeling bony to palpation.

The subscapularis bursa lies deep to the tendon in front of the neck of the scapula and usually communicates with the joint capsule of the shoulder. It is invariably extremely tender to palpation even when not inflamed.

Technique
- Patient sits supported with arm by side and held in 45° lateral rotation
- Identify the coracoid process. Move laterally to feel small protuberance of lesser tuberosity by passively rotating arm. Mark medial aspect of tuberosity
- Insert needle at this point, angling slightly laterally and touching bone at insertion for tendon, or in sagittal plane through tendon to enter the bursa
- Pepper solution into tendon insertion, or as a bolus deep to tendon into bursa

Aftercare
Relative rest for 1 week is advised, then progressive stretching and strengthening programme when pain-free. In sporting overuse injuries the cause should also be addressed.

Comments
Subscapularis bursitis and tendinitis are often difficult to differentiate. The bursa is implicated if there is more pain on the scarf test than on resisted medial rotation, and if there is even more than usual tenderness to palpation.

Alternative approaches
If the bursa and tendon are inflamed together they can both be infiltrated at the same time by peppering the tendon first and then going through it to infiltrate the bursa. The total dose is increased to 30 mg in total volume of 3 ml.

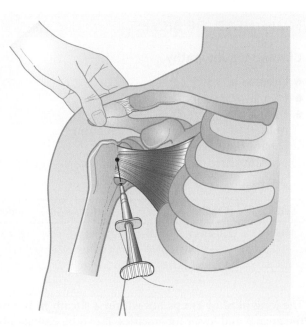

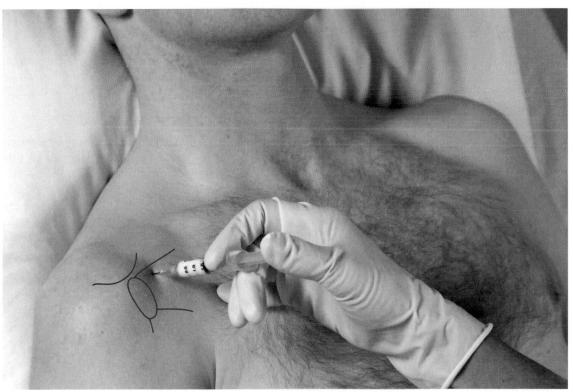

LONG HEAD OF BICEPS

Chronic tendinopathy

Causes and findings
- Overuse
- Pain anterior top of humerus
- Painful:
  resisted elbow flexion with supination
  passive shoulder extension
  occasional arc on shoulder elevation

Equipment

Syringe	Needle	Kenalog 40	Lidocaine	Total volume
1 ml	23G 1–1.25 inches (25–30 mm) Blue	10 mg	0.75 ml 2%	1 ml

Anatomy The long head of biceps lies within a sheath in the bicipital groove between the greater and lesser tuberosities. It can be palpated by getting the patient to contract the muscle under the palpating finger in the groove.

Technique
- Patient sits with supported elbow held at right angle
- Identify tender area of tendon
- Insert needle perpendicular to skin at highest part of tenderness, then angle downwards parallel to tendon
- Inject solution as a bolus between tendon and sheath

Aftercare Advise relative rest for 1 week then address the causes of the lesion.

Comments This lesion is commonly diagnosed but, in our experience, is quite rare. Palpation of what is normally a tender area can lead to a misdiagnosis of this tendinopathy, when it might be pain referred from the cervical spine, shoulder joint or rotator cuff lesion.

  If there is a sudden onset of pain on flexing, a distinct bulge can appear mid-humerus, indicating rupture of the long head of biceps. After the pain has subsided the patient is usually able to function normally because the short head is sufficient to take over flexion activities.

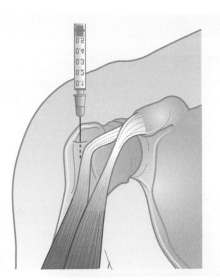

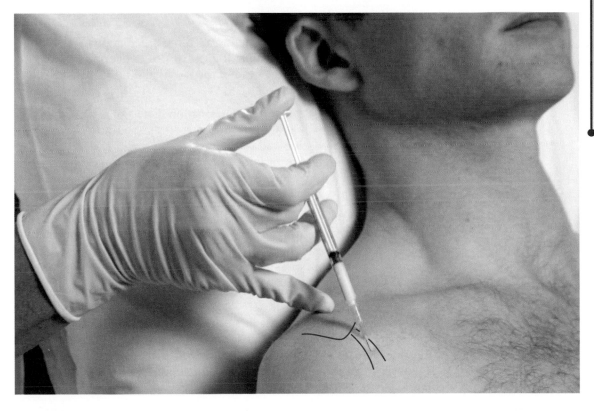

ELBOW JOINT

Acute or chronic capsulitis

Causes and findings
- Degenerative, inflammatory or traumatic arthropathies
- Occasionally heavy overuse, e.g. tennis, fencing
- Pain in and around elbow joint
- Painful limitation in the capsular pattern – *more*: loss of flexion than extension with a hard end feel

Equipment

Syringe	Needle	Kenalog 40	Lidocaine	Total volume
2 ml	23G 1.25 inches (30 mm) Blue	20 mg	1.5 ml 2%	2 ml

Anatomy The capsule of the elbow joint contains all three articulations – the radio-humeral, radioulnar and humeroulnar joints. The posterior approach into the small gap between the top of the head of the radius and the capitulum of the humerus is the safest and easiest.

Technique
- Patient sits with elbow supported in pronation at 45° of flexion
- Identify gap of joint line above head of radius posteriorly by passively moving elbow into flexion and extension
- Insert needle at mid-point of joint line parallel to the top of the head of radius, and penetrate capsule
- Inject solution as a bolus

Aftercare After a couple of days the patient should start increasing range of motion within the limits of pain using gentle stretching movements, especially into flexion. Passive mobilization techniques are effective in achieving full range but should be given with care in order not to further traumatize the joint.

Comments This is not a very common injection but may be useful after trauma or fracture of the radial head.

If the cause of the symptoms is one or more loose bodies within the joint, the treatment is mobilization under strong traction. If the range is improved by this but the pain persists, an injection may be considered.

Adolescents with loose bodies in the joint should be referred for surgical removal.

Alternative approaches If the joint is very degenerated, osteophytosis might be present around the joint margin, making entry with the needle more difficult. Deposition of a small amount of the solution into the capsule enables the clinician to 'walk' around the joint line with minimal discomfort to the patient. Some clinicians favour the posterior approach to the joint, inserting the needle at the top of the olecranon and angling obliquely distally.

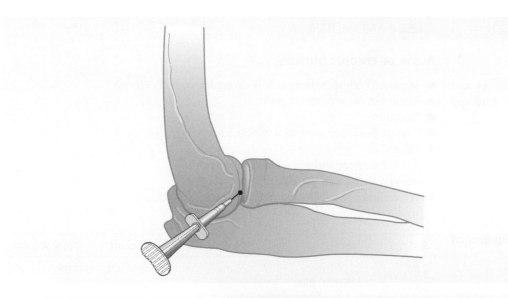

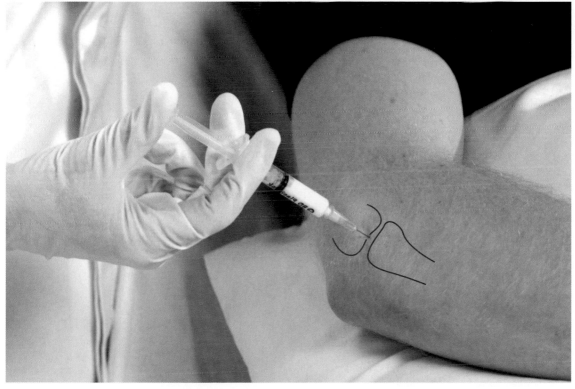

OLECRANON BURSA

Acute or chronic bursitis

Causes and findings
- Sustained compression or fall/direct blow onto elbow
- Rheumatoid arthritis or gout
- Infection
- Pain at posterior aspect of elbow joint
- Painful:
  passive flexion and sometimes extension
  resisted extension occasionally
- Tender area over bursa and often obvious swelling

Equipment

Syringe	Needle	Kenalog 40	Lidocaine	Total volume
2 ml	23G 1 inch (25 mm) Blue	20 mg	1.5 ml 2%	2 ml

Anatomy
The bursa lies subcutaneously at the posterior aspect of the elbow and is approximately the size of a golf ball.

Technique
- Patient sits with supported elbow at right angle
- Identify centre of tender area of bursa
- Insert needle into this point
- Inject solution as a bolus

Aftercare
Advise relative rest for 1 week, then resumption of normal activities avoiding leaning on elbow.

Comments
If swelling is present, always aspirate first. If suspicious fluid is withdrawn, infiltration should not be given until the aspirate has been investigated.

Occasionally a direct blow or fall can cause haemorrhagic bursitis. In these cases, the treatment should be immediate aspiration of all blood prior to infiltration.

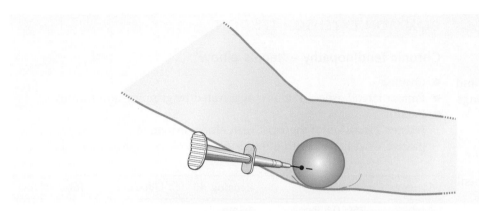

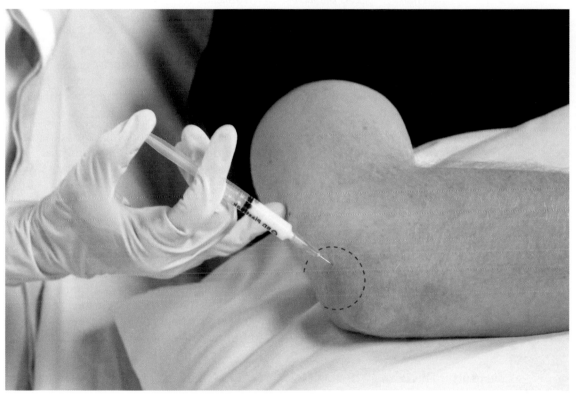

COMMON EXTENSOR TENDON

Chronic tendinopathy – 'tennis elbow'

Causes and findings
- Overuse
- Pain at lateral aspect of elbow aggravated by gripping and turning
- Painful:
  resisted extension of the wrist with elbow extended
  passive wrist flexion with ulnar deviation

Equipment

Syringe	Needle	Kenalog 40	Lidocaine	Total volume
1 ml	25G 0.5 inch (16 mm) Orange	10 mg	0.75 ml 2%	1 ml

Anatomy
Tennis elbow invariably occurs at the teno-osseous origin, or enthesis, of the common extensor tendon at the elbow. The tendon arises from the anterior facet of the lateral epicondyle, which is approximately the size of the little finger nail.

Technique
- Patient sits with supported elbow at right angle and forearm supinated
- Identify lateral point of epicondyle then move anteriorly onto facet
- Insert needle in line with cubital crease perpendicular to the facet to touch bone
- Pepper solution into tendon enthesis

Aftercare
The patient rests the elbow for 10 days. Any lifting must be done only with the palm facing upwards so that the flexors rather than the extensors are used; the causal activity must be avoided. When resisted extension is pain-free, two or three sessions of deep friction with a strong extension manipulation (Mill's manipulation) are given to prevent recurrence. Stretching of the extensors and a strengthening programme is then gradually introduced. If the cause was a racket sport, the weight, handle-size and stringing of the racket should be checked; as should the technique. Continuous static positions at work should be avoided.

Comments
This is a very common injectable lesion. Although the teno-osseous junction is the most usual site, the lesion can occur in the body of the tendon, in the muscle belly and at the origin of the extensor carpi radialis longus. Ignore tender trigger points in the body of the tendon, present in everyone, and place the needle exactly at the very small site of the lesion. 'Repetitive strain injury' can include true tennis elbow but neural stretching, relaxation techniques, cervical mobilization and postural advice might be effective if the tendon is clear.

One injection usually suffices but, if symptoms recur, a second injection can be given followed by the above routine 10 days later.

Alternative approaches
Sclerosant injection can be used, or tenotomy may be performed. Depigmentation and/or subcutaneous atrophy can occur in thin females, especially those with dark skins, and they should be informed of this before giving consent. Hydrocortisone should be used if the patient is concerned about these possible side-effects.

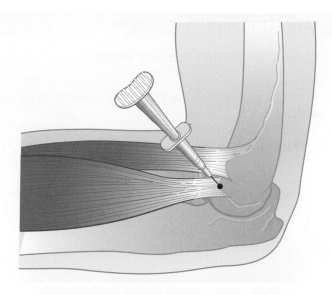

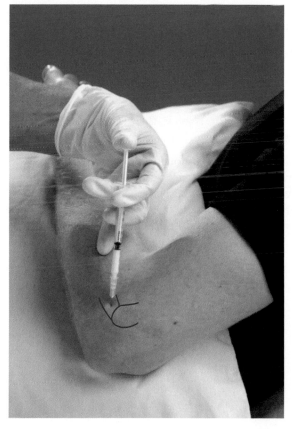

COMMON FLEXOR TENDON

Chronic tendinitis – 'golfer's elbow'

Causes and findings
- Overuse
- Pain at medial aspect of elbow aggravated by gripping and lifting
- Painful:
  resisted flexion of wrist
  occasionally resisted pronation of forearm

Equipment

Syringe	Needle	Kenalog 40	Lidocaine	Total volume
1 ml	25G 0.5 inch (16mm) Orange	10 mg	0.75 ml 2%	1 ml

Anatomy
The common flexor tendon at the elbow arises from the anterior facet on the medial epicondyle. It is approximately the size of the little finger nail at its teno-osseous origin.

Technique
- Patient sits with supported arm extended
- Identify facet lying anteriorly on medial epicondyle
- Insert needle perpendicular to facet and touch bone
- Pepper solution into tendon

Aftercare
Relative rest for 1 week, then stretching and strengthening exercises can be started.

Comments
Occasionally the lesion occurs at the musculotendinous junction, which is invariably a very tender point. Infiltration at this point might not be as effective but deep friction can be successful. This lesion is not as common as tennis elbow and less prone to recurrence, so follow-up treatment of deep friction and manipulation do not seem to be necessary.

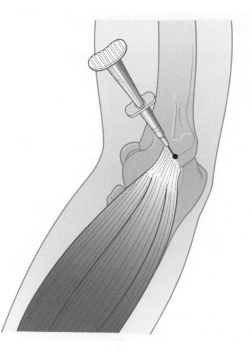

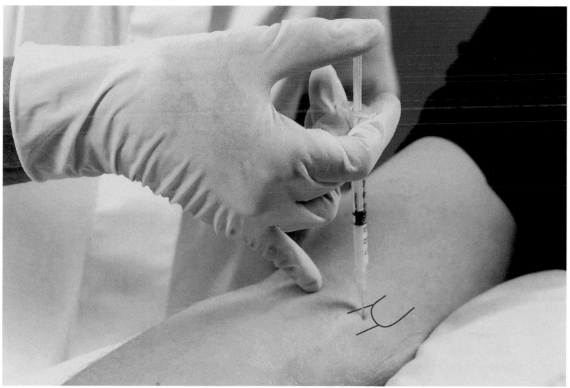

BICEPS TENDON INSERTION

Chronic tendinopathy or bursitis

Causes and findings
- Overuse
- Pain at front of elbow
- Painful:
  resisted flexion and supination of elbow
  plus full passive flexion, extension and pronation of elbow if bursa affected – a 'muddle' of signs

Equipment

Syringe	Needle	Kenalog 40	Lidocaine	Total volume
Tendon 1 ml Bursa 2ml	23G 1 inch (25 mm) Blue	Tendon 10mg Bursa 20mg	Tendon 0.75 ml 2% Bursa 1.5 ml 2%	Tendon 1 ml Bursa 2 ml

Anatomy
Although the biceps can be affected at any point along its length, the insertion into the radial tuberosity on the anteromedial aspect of the shaft of the radius is particularly vulnerable. A small bursa lies at this point and can be inflamed together with the tendon or on its own.

The insertion of the biceps is identified by following the path of the tendon distal to the cubital crease while the patient resists elbow flexion. The patient then relaxes the muscle and the tuberosity can be palpated on the ulnar side of the radius while passively pro- and supinating the forearm. The site is always very tender to palpation, even in the normal elbow.

Technique
- Patient lies face down with arm extended and palm flat on table. Fix humerus on table and passively fully pronate forearm. This brings the radial tuberosity round to face posteriorly
- Identify radial tuberosity two fingers distal to radial head
- Insert needle perpendicularly to touch bone
- Pepper solution into tendon or bolus into bursa, or both, as necessary

Aftercare
Rest for 1 week before beginning graded strengthening and stretching routine, followed by addressing the cause of the overuse.

Comments
Differentiation between bursitis and tendonopathy is often difficult. If there is more pain on passive flexion and pronation of the elbow than on resisted flexion, together with extreme sensitivity to palpation, the bursa is more suspect.

Alternative approaches
If a double lesion is suspected, infiltrate the bursa first and reassess 1 week later. The tendon can then be injected if necessary.

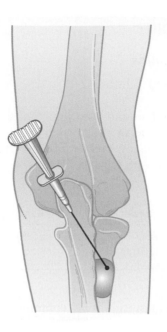

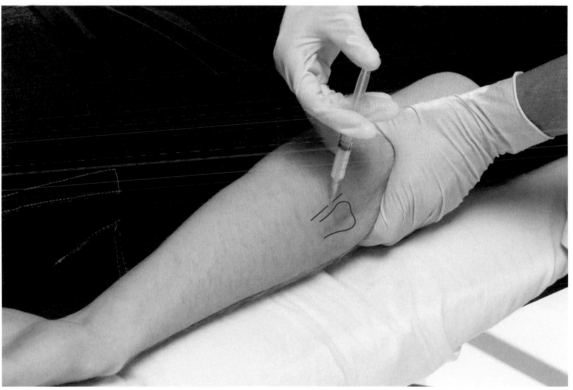

WRIST JOINT

Acute capsulitis

Causes and findings
- Rheumatoid arthritis
- Trauma
- Pain in and around wrist joint. There may also be heat, palpable synovial thickening and/or swelling
- Painful limitation in the capsular pattern – *equal*: loss of passive extension and flexion with hard end-feel

Equipment

Syringe	Needle	Kenalog 40	Lidocaine	Total volume
2 ml	23G 1.25 inches (30 mm) Blue	20 mg	1.5 ml 2%	2 ml

Anatomy
The wrist joint capsule is not continuous and has septa dividing it into separate compartments. For this reason it cannot be injected at one spot, but requires several areas of infiltration through one injection entry point.

Technique
- Patient places the hand palm down in some degree of wrist flexion
- Identify mid-carpus proximal to hollow dip of capitate
- Insert needle at mid-point of carpus
- Inject at different points across the dorsum of the wrist, both into the ligaments and also intracapsular where possible

Aftercare
The patient rests in a splint until the pain subsides and then begins gentle mobilizing exercises within the pain-free range. Wax baths can be most beneficial because the wax can be used as an exercise medium after being peeled off the hands.

Comments
This is a common area for injection in patients with rheumatoid arthritis.

Patients with other causes such as trauma, overuse or osteoarthritis usually respond well to a short period of pain-relieving modalities, medication and rest in a splint, followed by passive and active mobilization techniques. As in all cases of trauma, fracture, especially of the scaphoid, should be eliminated.

Alternative approaches
If the joint is badly affected and swollen, it might be necessary to use a longer needle to reach all around the area, or to inject at several points.

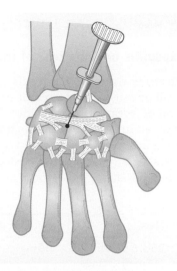

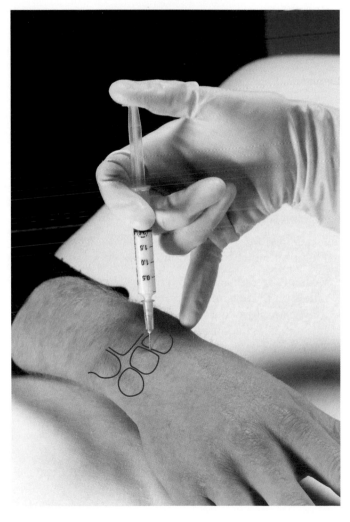

INFERIOR RADIOULNAR JOINT

Chronic capsulitis or acute tear of the meniscus

Causes and findings
- Osteoarthritis or rheumatoid arthritis
- Trauma: fall on outstretched hand or strong traction or twisting movement
- Pain at end of forearm on ulnar side
- Painful limitation in the capsular pattern: passive pronation and supination at end-range
- For meniscal tear: passive and resisted wrist flexion, with resisted and passive ulnar deviation, plus 'scoop' test (see below)

Equipment

Syringe	Needle	Kenalog 40	Lidocaine	Total volume
2 ml	25G 0.5 inch (16 mm) Orange	10 mg	1 ml 2%	1.25 ml

Anatomy The inferior radioulnar joint is an L-shaped joint about a finger's width in length and includes a triangular cartilage, which separates the ulna from the carpus. With the palm facing downwards, the joint runs one-third across the wrist just medial to the bump of the end of the ulna. The joint line is identified by gliding the ends of the radius and ulna against each other or by palpating the space between the styloid process of the ulna and the triquetral.

Technique
- Patient sits with hand palm down
- Identify styloid process of ulnar
- Insert needle just distal to styloid aiming transversely towards radius, passing through the ulnar collateral ligament to penetrate capsule
- Inject solution as a bolus

Aftercare Advise rest for 1 week with avoidance of flexion/ulnar deviation activities. Mobilization with distraction can be effective in meniscal tears.

Comments Tears of the cartilage are relatively common, especially after trauma such as falling on the outstretched hand, a traction injury or after Colles' fracture. The most pain-provoking test is the scoop test – compressing the supinated wrist into ulnar deviation and scooping it in a semi-circular movement towards flexion. The patient often complains of painful clicking and occasionally the wrist locks. Mobilization helps relieve the pain but an injection can be given in the acute phase. Often an explanation of the condition and reassurance, together with advice on avoidance, is sufficient.

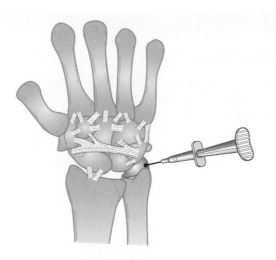

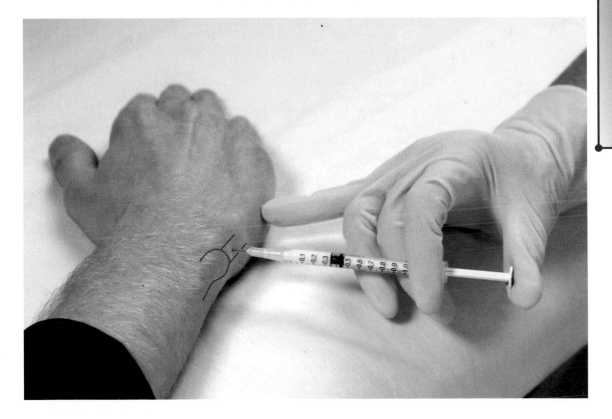

THUMB AND FINGER JOINTS

Acute or chronic capsulitis

Causes and findings
- Overuse or trauma
- Rheumatoid or degenerative arthritis
- Capsular pattern
- Thumb:
  painful and limited passive adduction of thumb backwards behind hand
  painful and limited passive extension and abduction
- Fingers:
  painful and limited extension with ulnar deviation at metacarpophalangeal joints
  painful and limited passive flexion at interphalangeal joints
  painful and limited passive extension at distal phalangeal joints

Equipment

Syringe	Needle	Kenalog 40	Lidocaine	Total volume
1 ml	25G 0.5 inch (16 mm) Orange	Thumb 10 mg Fingers 10 mg	Thumb 0.75 ml 2% Fingers 0.5 ml 2%	Thumb 1 ml Fingers 0.75 ml

Anatomy
The first metacarpal articulates with the trapezium. The easiest entry site is at the apex of the snuff-box on the dorsum of the wrist. The joint line is found by passively flexing and extending the thumb while palpating for the joint space between the two bones. The radial artery lies at the base of the snuff-box.

The distal thumb joint, and all finger joints can best be infiltrated from the medial or lateral aspect at the joint line.

Technique
- Patient rests hand in mid position with thumb up and traction is applied by patient
- Identify gap of joint space at apex of snuff box on dorsum of wrist
- Insert needle perpendicularly into gap
- Inject solution as a bolus

Aftercare
Tape the thumb using a spica technique, or tape two fingers together to splint them for a few days. Patient then begins gentle active and passive mobilizing exercise within pain-free range and is advised against overuse of the thumb or fingers. Dipping the fingers into warm wax baths and using the wax ball as an exercise tool can be beneficial.

Comments
Trapeziometacarpal joint capsulitis is a common lesion of older females and the results of infiltration are uniformly excellent. Often it is several years before a repeat injection is required, provided the patient does not grossly overuse the joint.

Alternative approaches
Infiltrating the thumb and finger joints can be difficult as osteophytosis will almost certainly be present. It is sometimes necessary to anaesthetize the capsule with some of the solution while trying to enter the joint. Gapping the side of the joint being entered also helps, and an even finer needle, such as 30G, can be used.

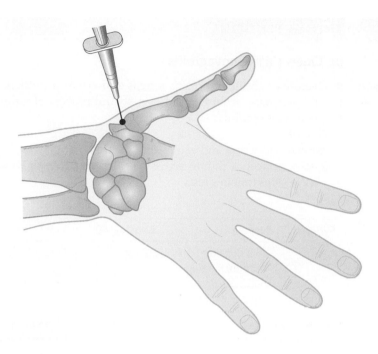

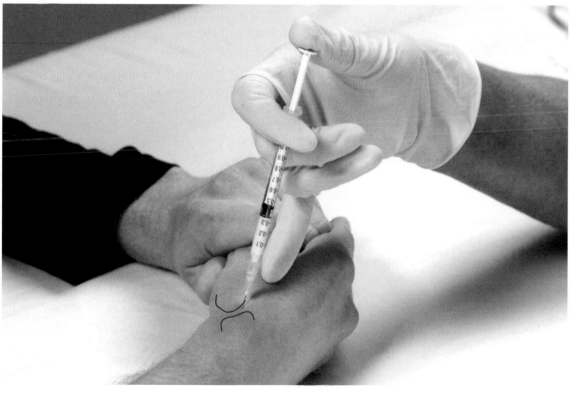

THUMB TENDONS

de Quervain's tenovaginitis

Causes and findings
- Overuse of abductor pollicis longus and extensor pollicis brevis
- Pain over base of thumb and over styloid process of radius
- Occasional crepitus
- Painful:
  resisted abduction and extension of thumb
  passive flexion of thumb across palm especially with wrist in ulnar deviation (Finklestein's test)

Equipment

Syringe	Needle	Kenalog 40	Lidocaine	Total volume
1 ml	25G 0.5 inch (16 mm) Orange	10 mg	0.75 ml 2%	1 ml

Anatomy
The abductor pollicis longus and extensor pollicis brevis usually run together in a single sheath on the radial side of the wrist. The styloid process is always tender so comparison should be made with the pain-free side. The two tendons can often be seen when the thumb is held in extension, or can be palpated at the base of the metacarpal. The aim is to slide the needle between the two tendons and deposit the solution within the sheath.

Technique
- Patient places hand vertically with thumb held in slight flexion
- Identify gap between the two tendons at base of first metacarpal
- Insert needle perpendicularly into gap then slide proximally between the tendons
- Inject solution as a bolus within tendon sheath

Aftercare
The patient should rest the hand for a week with taping of the tendons. This is followed by avoidance of the provoking activity and a graded strengthening regime if necessary.

Comments
Provided the wrist is not too swollen, a small sausage-shaped swelling can often be seen where the solution distends the tendon sheath.

Alternative approaches
This is an area where depigmentation or subcutaneous fat atrophy can occur, especially noticeable in dark-skinned thin females. Although recovery can take place, the results might be permanent. Patient should be warned of this possibility before giving their consent. The potential risk can be minimized by injecting with hydrocortisone.

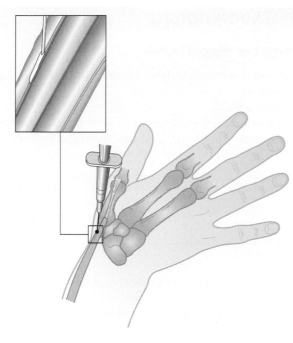

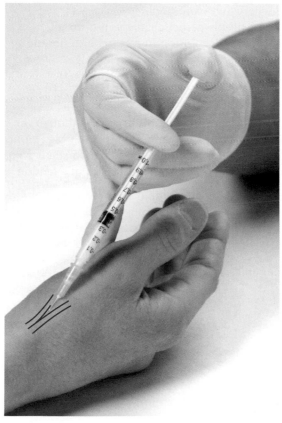

FLEXOR TENDON NODULE

Trigger finger or trigger thumb

Causes and findings
- Spontaneous onset: might have osteoarthritis or palpable ganglia in the fingers or hand
- Rheumatoid arthritis
- Painful clicking and sometimes locking of finger with inability to extend
- A tender nodule can be palpated usually at the base of the finger

Equipment

Syringe	Needle	Kenalog 40	Lidocaine	Total volume
1 ml	25G 0.5 inch (16mm) Orange	10mg	0.25 ml 2%	0.5 ml

Anatomy
Trigger finger is caused by enlargement of a nodule within the flexor tendon sheath, which then becomes inflamed and painful. It usually occurs at the joint lines where the tendon is tethered down by the ligaments.

Technique
- Patient places hand palm up
- Identify and mark nodule
- Insert needle perpendicularly into nodule
- Deposit half solution in a bolus into nodule
- Angle needle distally into sheath
- Deposit remaining solution into sheath

Aftercare
No particular restriction is placed on the patient's activities.

Comments
This injection is invariably effective. Although the nodule usually remains, it can continue to be asymptomatic indefinitely, but recurrence can be treated with a further injection. Occasionally a slight pop is felt as the needle penetrates the nodule. When the needle is in a tendon, a rubbery resistance is felt.

Alternative approaches
Some clinicians insert the needle alone first and then ask the patient to flex the finger. If the needle moves, this proves that the correct site has been reached and the syringe may then be attached. As this involves delay and discomfort to the patient, we recommend the method above.

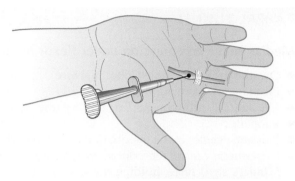

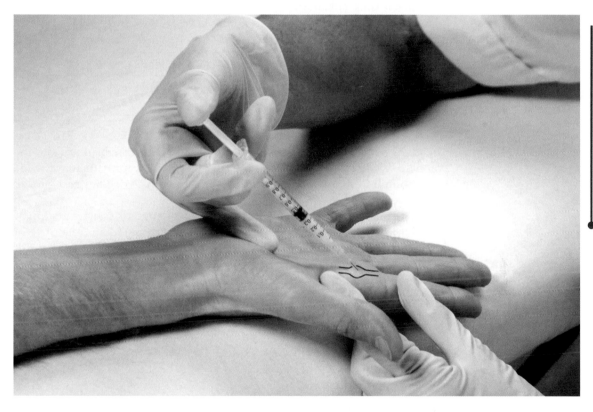

CARPAL TUNNEL

Median nerve compression under flexor retinaculum

Causes and findings
- Overuse or trauma, post-Colles' fracture
- Pregnancy, hypothyroidism, acromegaly
- Rheumatoid arthritis, psoriatic arthropathy
- Idiopathic
- Pins and needles in the distribution of the median nerve, especially at night
- Paraesthesia can be reproduced by tapping the median nerve at the wrist (Tinnel's sign) or by holding the wrist in full flexion for 30 seconds and then releasing (Phalen's sign). Longstanding median nerve compression may cause flattening of the thenar eminence

Equipment

Syringe	Needle	Kenalog 40	Lidocaine	Total volume
1 ml	23G 1.25 inches (30 mm) Blue	20 mg	Nil	0.5 ml

Anatomy
The flexor retinaculum of the wrist attaches to four sites: the pisiform and the scaphoid, the hook of hamate and the trapezium. It is approximately as wide as the thumb from proximal to distal and the proximal edge lies at the distal wrist crease.

The median nerve lies immediately under the palmaris longus tendon at the mid-point of the wrist, and medial to the flexor carpi radialis tendon. Not every patient will have a palmaris longus so ask the patient to press tip of thumb onto tip of little finger; the crease seen at mid-point of the palm points to where the median nerve should run.

Technique
- Patient places hand palm up
- Identify point midway along proximal wrist crease, between flexor carpi radialis and median nerve
- Insert needle at this point then angle it 45°. Slide distally until needle end lies under mid-point of retinaculum
- Inject solution in bolus

Aftercare
The patient rests for 1 week and then resumes normal activities. A night splint helps in the early stages after the infiltration and the patient is advised to avoid sleeping with the wrists held in full flexion – the 'dormouse' position.

Comments
No local anaesthetic is used here because the main symptom is paraesthesia, not pain, and it is not advisable to increase the pressure within the tunnel. Care should be taken to avoid inserting the needle too vertically, when it will go into bone, or too horizontally, when it will enter the retinaculum. If the patient experiences pins and needles, the needle is in the median nerve and must be withdrawn slightly and repositioned. Although one injection is often successful, recurrences do occur. Further injections can be given if some relief was obtained, but if the symptoms still recur surgery may be required.

Alternative approach
The injection can be equally well performed by inserting the needle between the median nerve and the flexor tendons, using the same dose and volume.

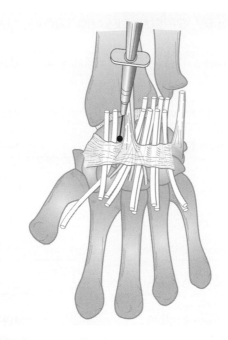

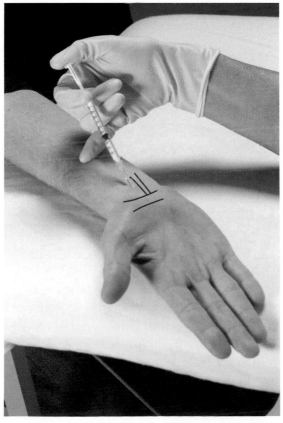

SUMMARY OF SUGGESTED UPPER LIMB DOSES

Syringe	Needle	Kenalog 40	Lidocaine	Total volume
Shoulder				
Shoulder joint 5 ml	Green 1.5 or 2 inches	40 mg	4 ml 1%	5 ml
Suprascapular nerve 1 ml	Green 1.75 inches	20 mg	Nil	0.5 ml
Acromioclavicular joint 1 ml	Orange 0.5 inch	10 mg	0.75 ml 2%	1 ml
Sternoclavicular joint 1 ml	Orange 0.5 inch	10 mg	0.75 ml 2%	1 ml
Subacromial bursa 5 ml	Green 1.25 inches	20 mg	4.5 ml 1%	5 ml
Supraspinatus tendon 1 ml	Orange 0.5 inch	10 mg	0.75 ml 2%	1 ml
Infraspinatus tendon 2 ml	Blue 1.25 inches	20 mg	1.5 ml 2%	2 ml
Subscapularis tendon/bursa 1 ml/2 ml	Blue 1.25 inches/ Green 2 inches	10/20 mg	0.75/1.5 ml 2%	1 ml/2 ml
Long head of biceps 1 ml	Blue 1–1.25 inches	10 mg	0.75 ml 2%	1 ml
Elbow				
Elbow joint 2 ml	Blue 1.25 inches	20 mg	1.5 ml 2%	2 ml
Olecranon bursa 2 ml	Blue 1 inch	20 mg	1.5 ml 2%	2 ml
Common extensor tendon 1 ml	Orange 0.5 inch	10 mg	0.75 ml 2%	1 ml
Common flexor tendon 1 ml	Orange 0.5 inch	10 mg	0.75 ml 2%	1 ml
Biceps tendon/bursa 1 ml/2 ml	Blue 1 inch	10 mg/20 mg	0.75/1.5 ml 2%	1 ml/2 ml
Wrist and hand				
Wrist joint 2 ml	Blue 1.25 inches	20 mg	1.5 ml 2%	2 ml
Inferior radio-ulnar joint 2 ml	Orange 0.5 inch	10 mg	1 ml 2%	1.25 ml
Thumb and finger joints 1 ml	Orange 0.5 inch	10 mg	0.75/0.5 ml 2%	1 ml/0.75 ml
Thumb tendons 1 ml	Orange 0.5 inch	10 mg	0.75 ml 2%	1 ml
Flexor tendon nodule 1 ml	Orange 0.5 inch	10 mg	0.25 ml 2%	0.5 ml
Carpal tunnel 1 ml	Blue 1.25 inches	20 mg	Nil	0.5 ml

SECTION 3

INJECTION TECHNIQUES OF THE LOWER LIMB

Finger measurements are from the patient, not the clinician.

Section 3

INFECTION
TECHNIQUES OF

ASSESSMENT OF THE LOWER LIMB

Hip tests

Supine	Passive	lateral rotation
		medial rotation
		flexion
		abduction
		adduction
	Resisted	flexion
		abduction
		adduction
Prone	Passive	extension
	Resisted	lateral rotation
		medial rotation
		knee extension
		knee flexion

Hip capsular pattern: most loss of medial rotation, less of flexion and abduction, least of extension

Knee tests

Passive	flexion	Draw test	
	extension	Glide test	
	valgus	Meniscal tests	
	varus	Resisted	extension
	lateral rotation		flexion
	medial rotation		

Knee capsular pattern: more loss of flexion than extension

Ankle tests

Passive	dorsiflexion
	plantarflexion
	eversion
	inversion

Forefoot tests

Passive	abduction
	adduction
	extension
	flexion

Subtalar tests

Calcaneal abduction	pronation
Calcaneal adduction	supination

Muscle tests

Resisted	dorsiflexion
	plantarflexion
	eversion
	inversion

Foot capsular patterns
Ankle: More loss of plantarflexion than dorsiflexion
Subtalar joint: More loss of adduction
Forefoot: Loss of adduction, dorsiflexion and supination
Big toe: More loss of extension than flexion
Other toes: More loss of flexion than extension

SECTION 3

HIP JOINT

Acute capsulitis

Causes and findings
- Osteoarthritis, rheumatoid arthritis or traumatic capsulitis with night pain and severe radiating pain no longer responding to physiotherapy
- May be on waiting list for surgery
- Buttock, groin and/or anterior thigh pain
- Painful limitation in capsular pattern – most: loss of medial rotation; less: loss of flexion and abduction; least: loss of extension
- Hard end-feel on passive testing

Equipment

Syringe	Needle	Kenalog 40	Lidocaine	Total volume
5 ml	22G 3.5 inches (90 mm) Spinal	40 mg	4 ml 1%	5 ml

Anatomy
The hip joint capsule attaches to the base of the surgical neck of the femur. Therefore, if the needle is inserted into the neck, the solution will be deposited within the capsule. The safest and easiest approach is from the lateral aspect.

The greater trochanter is triangular in shape with a sharp angulation inwards or the apex overhanging the neck. This part is difficult to palpate, especially on patients with excessive adipose tissue, so insert needle at least a thumb's width proximal to the most prominent part of the trochanter.

Technique
- Patient lies on pain-free side with lower leg flexed and upper leg straight and resting on pillow so that it lies horizontal
- Identify apex of greater trochanter with finger while passively abducting patient's upper leg
- Insert needle perpendicularly about a thumb's width proximal to palpable apex of trochanter until it touches the neck of femur
- Inject solution as a bolus

Aftercare
Patient gradually increases pain-free activity maintaining range with a home stretching routine but limits weight-bearing exercise.

Comments
The lateral approach to the hip joint is both simple and safe. It is not necessary to do the technique under fluoroscopy and the procedure is not painful. There is usually no sensation of penetrating the capsule. This injection is usually given to patients who are on a waiting list for surgery, but the joint should not be injected within at least 6 weeks of surgery because reduced immunity could result in greater possible risk of infection. It is usually successful in giving temporary pain relief and can, if necessary, be repeated at intervals of no less than 3 months. An annual X-ray monitors degenerative changes.

Alternative approaches
For large patients the total volume can be increased to 8–10 ml. Forty mg Adcortyl, giving 4 ml of volume, might be the preferred steroid here. For large individuals, a longer spinal needle might be required.

During the early stages of the degenerative process, when the pain is local, there is minimal night pain and end feels are still elastic with reasonably good function, physiotherapy can be effective.

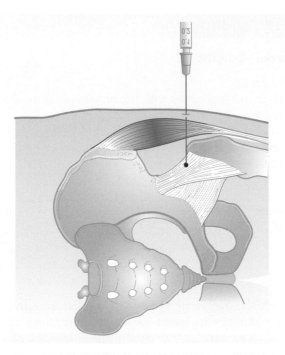

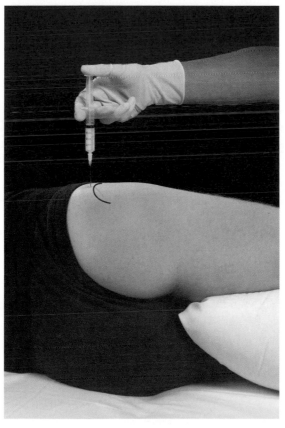

GLUTEAL BURSA

Chronic bursitis

Causes and findings
- Overuse
- Pain and tenderness over the upper lateral quadrant of the buttock
- Painful:
  passive flexion, abduction and adduction
  resisted abduction and extension
- End-feel normal

Equipment

Syringe	Needle	Kenalog 40	Lidocaine	Total volume
5 ml	22G 3.5 inches (90 mm) Spinal	40 mg	4 ml 1%	5 ml

Anatomy
The gluteal bursae are variable in number, size and shape. They can lie deep to the gluteal muscles on the blade of the ilium and also between the layers of the three muscles. The painful site guides the placement of the needle but comparison between the two sides is essential as this area is always tender.

Technique
- Patient lies on unaffected side with lower leg extended and upper leg flexed
- Identify and mark centre of tender area in upper outer quadrant of buttock
- Insert needle perpendicular to skin until it touches bone of ilium
- Inject solution in areas of no resistance while moving needle in a circular manner out towards surface – imagine the needle walking up a spiral staircase

Aftercare
The patient must avoid overusing the leg for a week and can then gradually resume normal activities. Addressing any muscle tightness or imbalance and retraining in the causative sporting activity is necessary.

Comments
There are no major blood vessels or nerves in the area of the bursae so the injection is safe. Feeling for a loss of resistance beneath and within the glutei guides the clinician in depositing the fluid.

Pain referring from the lumbar spine or sacroiliac joint can often be mistaken for gluteal bursitis. The mere presence of tenderness mid-buttock, normal in most individuals, should not be considered diagnostic of an inflamed bursa.

Alternative approaches
For large individuals, a longer spinal needle might be required.

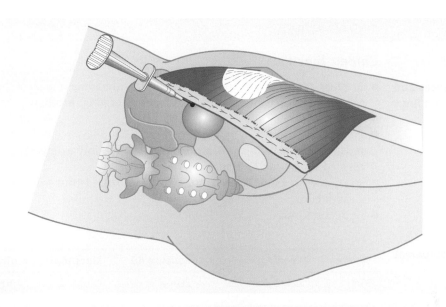

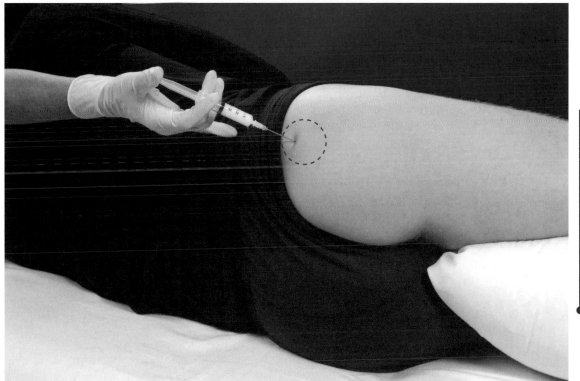

PSOAS BURSA

Chronic bursitis

Causes and findings
- Overuse – especially sports or activities involving repeated hip flexion movements, e.g. hurdling, ballet, javelin throwing, football
- Pain in groin
- Painful:
  passive flexion, adduction, abduction and possibly extension
  resisted flexion and adduction
  scoop test – passive semicircular compression of femur from full flexion to adduction
- End-feel normal

Equipment

Syringe	Needle	Kenalog 40	Lidocaine	Total volume
5 ml	22G 3.5 inches (90 mm) Spinal	20 mg	4 ml 1%	4.5 ml

Anatomy
The psoas bursa lies between the iliopsoas tendon and the anterior aspect of the capsule over the neck of the femur. It is situated deep to three major structures in the groin – the femoral vein, artery and nerve, lying at the level of the inguinal ligament. For this reason, careful placement of the needle is essential. Following the instructions below ensures that the needle will pass obliquely beneath the neurovascular bundle.

Technique
- Patient lies supine
- Identify femoral pulse at mid-point of inguinal ligament. Mark a point three fingers distally and three fingers laterally. The entry point lies in direct line with the anterior superior iliac spine and passes through the medial edge of the sartorius muscle
- Insert needle at this point and aim 45° cephalad and 45° medially. Visualize the needle sliding under the three major vessels through the psoas tendon until point touches bone on anterior aspect of neck of femur
- Withdraw slightly and inject as bolus deep to tendon

Aftercare
Absolute avoidance of the activities that irritated the bursa must be maintained for at least 1 week, then stretching of hip extension and muscle-balancing programme is initiated.

Comments
Although this injection might appear intimidating to the clinician at the first attempt, the approach outlined above is safe and effective. Very occasionally it is possible to catch a lateral branch of the femoral nerve and temporarily lose power in the quadriceps. If the patient complains of a tingling or burning pain during the process, reposition the needle before depositing solution.

Differential diagnoses include local lesions such as hip joint pathology, adductor strain, hernia, abdominal muscle sprain, cutaneous nerve entrapment, pubic symphysis, testicular disease, fracture and referred symptoms from lumbar spine, sacroiliac joint and genitourinary organs. Suspicion of any

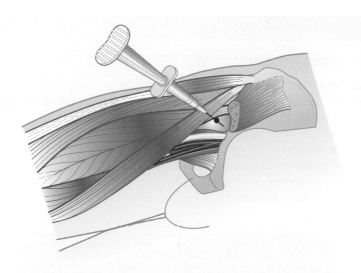

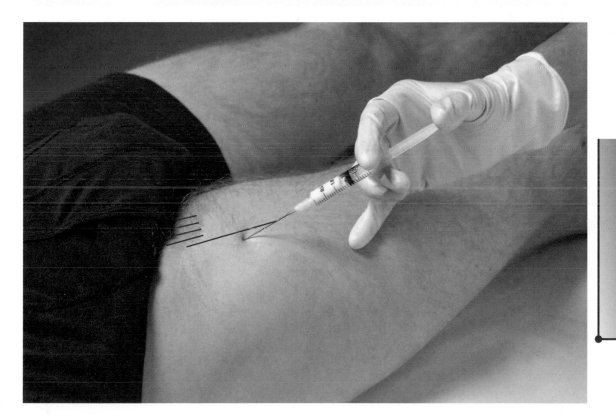

of these should be maintained until the clinician is satisfied of the cause of the symptoms. If in doubt, a diagnostic injection of local anaesthetic alone is advisable.

Alternative approaches For large individuals, a longer spinal needle might be required.

TROCHANTERIC BURSA

Acute or chronic bursitis

Causes and findings
- Usually a direct blow or fall onto hip
- Occasionally overuse or, in the thin elderly patient, lying on the same side every night, usually on a hard mattress
- Pain and tenderness over greater trochanter
- Painful:
  passive abduction, adduction and possibly flexion and extension of the hip
  resisted abduction

Equipment

Syringe	Needle	Kenalog 40	Lidocaine	Total volume
2 ml	23G 1.25 inches (30 mm) Blue	20 mg	1.5 ml 2%	2 ml

Anatomy
The trochanteric bursa lies over the greater trochanter of the femur. It is approximately the size of a golf ball and is usually tender to palpation.

Technique
- Patient lies on unaffected side with lower leg flexed and upper leg extended
- Identify and mark tender area over greater trochanter
- Insert needle perpendicularly at centre of tender area and touch bone of greater trochanter
- Inject by feeling for area of lack of resistance and introduce fluid there as a bolus

Aftercare
Patient should avoid overuse for 1 week and then gradually return to normal activity. If the cause is lying on a hard mattress, the trochanter can be padded with a large circle of sticky felt. A change of lying position is encouraged and the mattress might need to be changed. Stretching of the iliotibial band can also help.

Comments
A fall or direct blow onto the trochanter will often cause a haemorrhagic bursitis. This calls for immediate aspiration of blood prior to the infiltration.

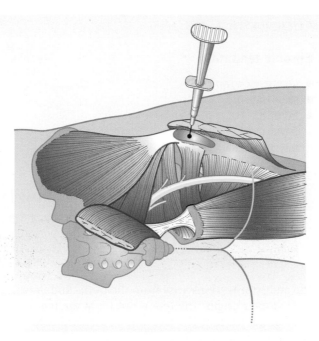

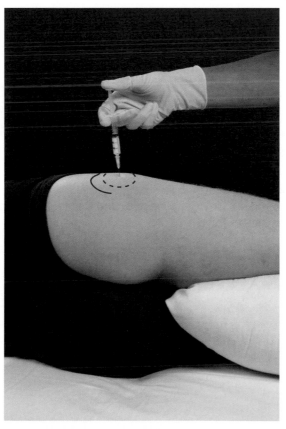

ADDUCTOR TENDONS

Chronic tendinitis

Causes and findings
- Overuse or trauma
- Pain in groin
- Painful:
  resisted adduction
  passive abduction

Equipment

Syringe	Needle	Kenalog 40	Lidocaine	Total volume
2 ml	23G 1.25 inches (30 mm) Blue	20 mg	1.5 ml 2%	2 ml

Anatomy
The adductor tendons arise from the pubis and are approximately two fingers wide at their origin. The lesion can lie at the teno-osseous junction or in the body of the tendon. The technique described is for the more common site at the teno-osseous junction.

Technique
- The patient lies supine with leg slightly abducted and laterally rotated
- Identify and mark the origin of the tendon
- Insert needle into tendon, angle towards pubis and touch bone
- Pepper solution into teno-osseous junction

Aftercare
Rest for at least 1 week then start a graduated stretching and strengthening programme. Deep friction massage may be used as well to mobilize the scar.

Comments
Sprain of these tendons is commonly thought to cause 'groin strain'. However, there are many alternative causes of pain in the groin (see psoas bursa technique) and these should be eliminated carefully.

Alternative approaches
For the less common site at the body of the tendon, the solution is peppered into the tender area in the body, but deep friction massage and stretching may be more effective here.

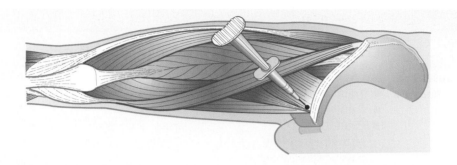

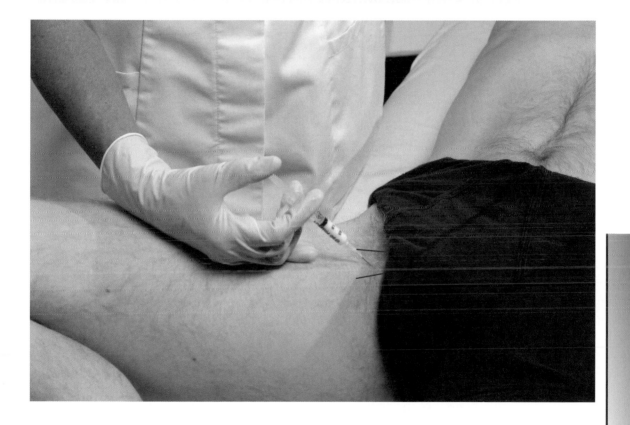

HAMSTRINGS – ORIGIN

Chronic tendinitis or acute or chronic ischial bursitis

Causes and findings
- Overuse – such as prolonged riding on horse or bicycle, or running
- Trauma – fall onto buttock, or sudden acceleration, kicking
- Pain in buttock
- Painful:
  resisted extension
  passive straight leg raise
- Very tender over ischial tuberosity

Equipment

Syringe	Needle	Kenalog 40	Lidocaine	Total volume
2 ml	21G 2 inches (50 mm) Green	20 mg	1.5 ml 2%	2 ml

Anatomy
The hamstrings have a common origin arising from the ischial tuberosity. The tendon is approximately three fingers wide here. The ischial bursa lies between the gluteus maximus and the bone of the ischial tuberosity.

Technique
- Patient lies on unaffected side with lower leg straight and upper leg flexed
- Identify ischial tuberosity and mark tendon lying immediately distal
- Insert needle into mid-point of tendon and angle up toward tuberosity to touch bone
- Pepper solution into teno-osseous junction of tendon or inject as bolus into bursa

Aftercare
Avoidance of precipitating activities such as sitting on hard surfaces or prolonged running is maintained for at least a week and then graduated stretching and strengthening programme is started.

Comments
Tendinitis and bursitis can occur together at this site, in which case a larger volume is drawn up and both lesions infiltrated. As usual, it is difficult to differentiate between the two lesions, but if there is a history of a fall or friction overuse and extreme tenderness at the tuberosity, bursitis is suspected.

Occasionally, haemorrhagic bursitis can occur as a result of a hard fall. Aspiration of the blood is then performed prior to infiltration.

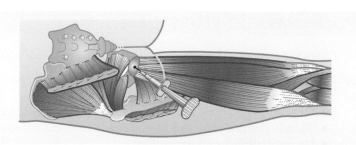

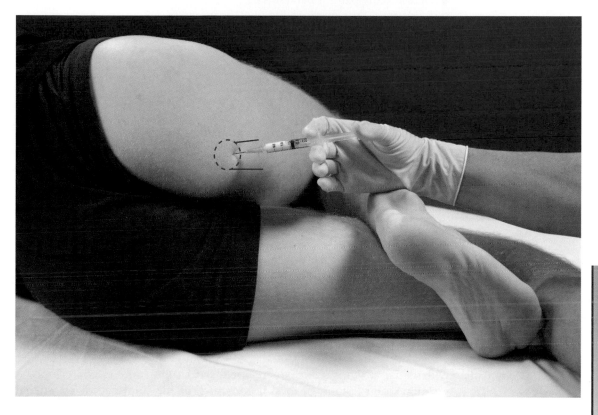

LATERAL CUTANEOUS NERVE

Meralgia paraesthetica

Causes and findings
- Entrapment neuropathy due to compression of the lateral cutaneous nerve of the thigh
- Obesity, pregnancy or prolonged static flexed positions
- Sharply defined oval area of numbness over anterolateral thigh
- Occasionally painful paraesthesia
- Tenderness over nerve at inguinal ligament or where the nerve emerges through the fascia

Equipment

Syringe	Needle	Kenalog 40	Lidocaine	Total volume
1 ml	21G 2 inches (50 mm) Green	20 mg	Nil	0.5 ml

Anatomy The lateral cutaneous nerve of the thigh arises from the outer border of the psoas and crosses over the iliacus. It passes under or through the inguinal ligament, through the femoral fascia and emerges superficially about 10 cm distal and in line with the anterior superior iliac spine.

Technique
- Patient lies supine
- Identify tender area at inguinal ligament or at distal point in thigh
- Inject as bolus around compressed nerve, avoiding nerve itself

Aftercare Removing the cause is of prime importance, i.e. losing weight, avoiding tight clothing, correcting sitting posture. If the patient is pregnant the compression might be from the growing fetus, and symptoms will normally abate after delivery.

Comments Differential diagnoses include referred symptoms from lumbar spine or sacroiliac joint lesions, or local lesions such as hip joint pathology, arterial claudication, herpes zoster.

As with other nerve compression injections, the nerve itself must not be injected. If the patient reports increased tingling or burning pain, the needle point should be moved before the steroid is injected.

Alternative approach This lesion often spontaneously resolves. Advice on avoidance of compression and reassurance as to the nature and normal outcome of the condition might be all that is required.

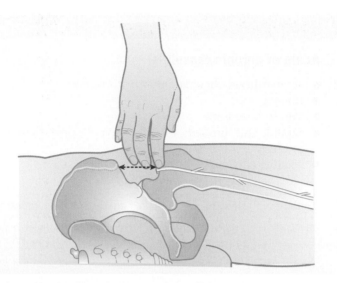

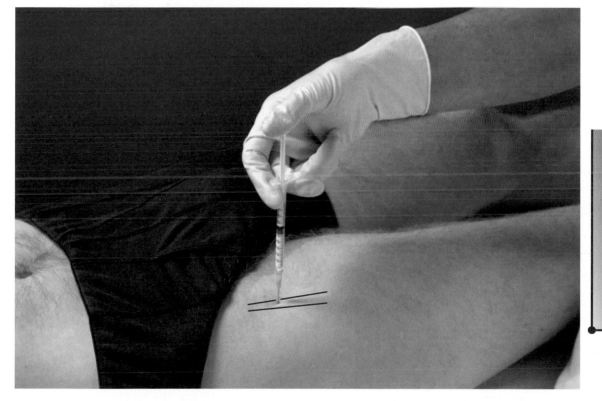

KNEE JOINT

Acute or chronic capsulitis

Causes and findings
- Osteoarthritis, rheumatoid arthritis or gout
- Trauma
- Pain in knee joint
- Painful and limited: more passive flexion than extension with hard end-feel
- Possible effusion

Equipment

Syringe	Needle	Kenalog 40	Lidocaine	Total volume
5–10 ml	21G 1.5 inches (40 mm) Green	40 mg	4 ml 1%– 9 ml 0.5%	5–10 ml

Anatomy   The knee joint has a potential capacity of approximately 120 ml in the average-sized adult. The capsule is lined with synovium, which is convoluted and so has a large surface area; in the large knee, therefore, more volume will be required to bathe all the surface. Plicae, which are bands of synovium, might exist within the joint and can also become inflamed. The suprapatellar pouch is a continuum of the synovial capsule and there are many bursae around the joint.

Technique
- Patient sits with knee supported in extension
- Identify and mark medial edge of patella
- Insert needle and angle laterally and slightly upwards under patella
- Inject solution as bolus or aspirate if required

Aftercare   The patient avoids undue weight-bearing activity for at least 1 week and is then given strengthening and mobilizing exercises to continue at home. One study indicated that total bed rest for 24 hours after injection in rheumatoid knees showed better results; however, the rest involved a hospital stay, which would not be cost effective.

Comments   The injection will give temporary relief from pain and, provided the knee is not overused, this can last for some time. Repeat injections can be given at intervals of not less than 3 months with an annual X-ray to monitor joint degeneration. As with the hip joint, the patient might be awaiting surgery; the injection should not be given for at least 6 weeks prior to this.

Alternative approaches   There are several ways to infiltrate or aspirate the knee joint – through the 'eyes of the knee', the supralateral approach into the suprapatella pouch just above the lateral pole of the patella, laterally at mid-point of patella or the medial approach as shown here. One study showed that there was more successful intra-articular placement using the lateral patella approach than through the 'eyes of the knee', but did not compare the lateral with this medial approach. The advantage of this approach is that there is normally plenty of space to insert the needle between the medial condyle and the patella, where even small amounts of effusion can be aspirated. The same approach can be used whether infiltrating or aspirating serous fluid or blood.

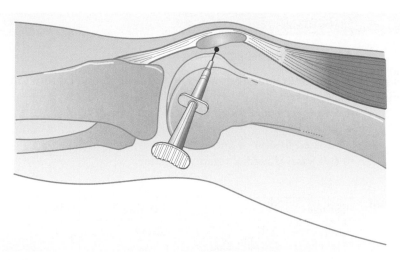

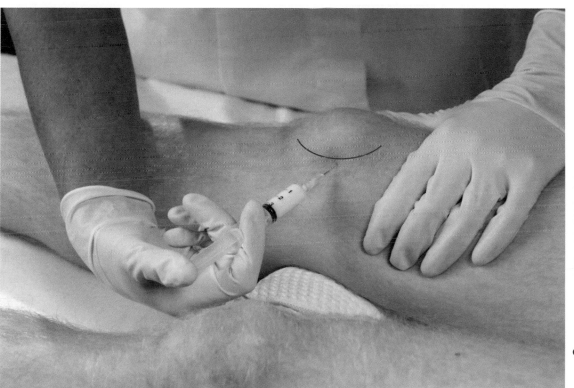

SECTION 3

For larger volumes, 40 mg Adcortyl, giving 4 ml of volume, might be the preferred steroid with less local anaesthetic. Hyalgen or similar substances can also be injected here but are more expensive than corticosteroids and do not appear to have longer-lasting benefits.

SUPERIOR TIBIOFIBULAR JOINT

Acute or chronic capsulitis

Causes and findings
- Usually trauma such as a fall with forced medial rotation and varus on a flexed knee
- Pain over lateral side of knee
- Painful:
  resisted flexion of knee
  full passive medial rotation of knee

Equipment

Syringe	Needle	Kenalog 40	Lidocaine	Total volume
2 ml	23G 1 inch (25 mm) Blue	20 mg	1 ml 2%	1.5 ml

Anatomy
The superior tibiofibular joint line runs medially from superior to inferior. The anterior approach is safer as the peroneal nerve lies posterior to the joint.

Technique
- Patient sits with knee at right angle
- Identify head of fibula and mark joint line medial to it
- Insert needle at mid-point of joint line and aim obliquely laterally to penetrate capsule
- Deposit solution in bolus

Aftercare
Advise relative rest for at least 1 week and then resumption of normal activities. Strengthening of the biceps femoris might be necessary.

Comments
Occasionally the joint is subluxed and has to be manipulated before infiltration. The condition also occasionally occurs after severe ankle sprain.

Alternative approach
The unstable joint can be treated with sclerotherapy.

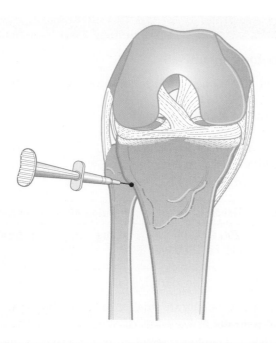

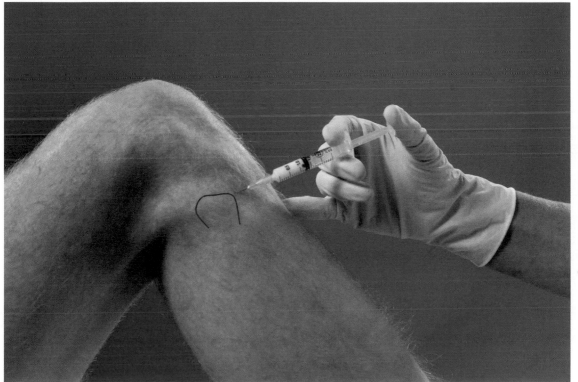

CORONARY LIGAMENTS

Ligamentous sprain

Causes and findings
- Trauma – a strong forced rotation of the knee with or without meniscal tear
- Pain usually at medial joint line
- Painful:
  passive lateral rotation
  possibly meniscal tests

Equipment

Syringe	Needle	Kenalog 40	Lidocaine	Total volume
1 ml	25G 0.5 inch (16 mm) Orange	10 mg	0.75 ml 2%	1 ml

Anatomy
The coronary ligaments are small thin fibrous bands attaching the menisci to the tibial plateaux.

The medial ligament is more usually affected. It can be found by placing the foot on the table with the knee at right angles and turning the foot into lateral rotation. This brings the tibial plateau into prominence and the tender area is sought by pressing in and down onto the plateau.

Technique
- Patient sits with knee at right angle and planted foot laterally rotated
- Identify and mark tender area on tibial plateau
- Insert needle vertically down onto plateau
- Pepper all along tender area

Aftercare
Early mobilizing exercise to full range of motion without pain is started immediately.

Comments
This lesion is commonly misdiagnosed; apparent meniscal tears, anterior cruciate sprain and patellofemoral joint lesions might be simple coronary ligament sprains.

Alternative approaches
These ligaments usually respond extremely well to deep friction massage – it is not uncommon to cure the symptoms in one session. The injection should be kept for where the friction treatment is not available or where the pain is too intense to allow the pressure of the finger.

Tear or subluxation of the meniscus should be treated first by manipulation.

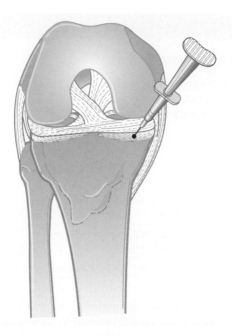

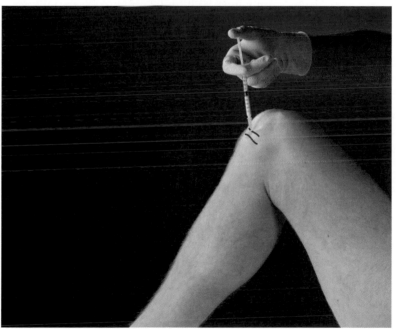

MEDIAL COLLATERAL LIGAMENT

Acute or chronic sprain

Causes and findings
- Trauma – typically flexion, valgus and lateral rotation of the knee as in a fall while skiing
- Pain at medial joint line of knee
- Painful:
  passive valgus
  passive lateral rotation of the knee

Equipment

Syringe	Needle	Kenalog 40	Lidocaine	Total volume
2 ml	23G 1.25 inches (30 mm) Blue	20 mg	1 ml 2%	1.5 ml

Anatomy
The medial collateral ligament of the knee passes distally from the medial condyle of the femur to the medial aspect of the shaft of the tibia and is approximately a hand's width long and a good two fingers wide at the joint line. It is difficult to palpate the ligament as it is so thin and is part of the joint capsule. It is usually sprained at the joint line.

Technique
- Patient lies with knee supported and slightly flexed
- Identify and mark medial joint line and tender area of ligament
- Insert needle at mid-point of tender area. Do not penetrate right through joint capsule
- Pepper solution along width of ligament in two rows

Aftercare
Gentle passive and active movement within the pain-free range is started immediately.

Comments
Occasionally the distal or proximal end of the ligament is affected, so the solution should be deposited there.

Alternative approaches
Sprain of this ligament rarely needs to be injected, as early physiotherapeutic treatment with ice, massage and mobilization is very effective. The injection approach can be used when this treatment is not available or the patient is in a great deal of pain.

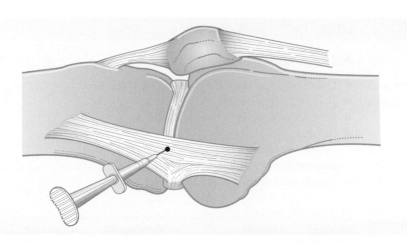

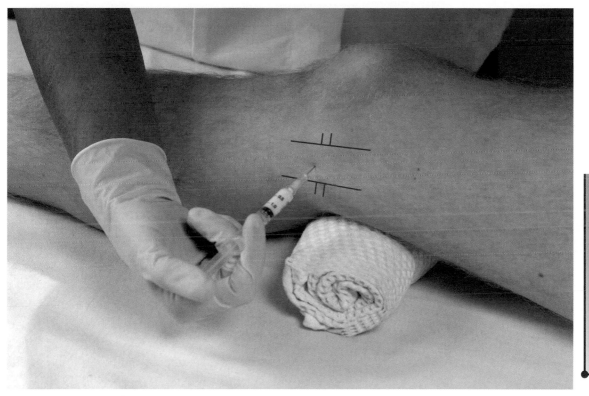

INFRAPATELLAR BURSA

Acute or chronic bursitis

Causes and findings
- Overuse –long distance running or prolonged kneeling
- Trauma – direct blow or fall
- Pain anterior knee below patella
- Painful:
  resisted extension of knee
  passive flexion of knee
- Tenderness at mid-point of patella tendon

Equipment

Syringe	Needle	Kenalog 40	Lidocaine	Total volume
2 ml	23G 1.25 inches (30 mm) Blue	20 mg	1.5 ml 2%	2 ml

Anatomy There are two infrapatellar bursae – one lies superficial and one deep to the tendon. In a small study it was found that the infrapatellar bursa consistently lay posterior to the distal third of the tendon and was slightly wider; a fat pad apron extends from the retropatellar fat pad to partially compartmentalize the bursa. The technique described is for the deep bursa, which is more commonly affected.

Technique
- Patient sits with leg extended and knee supported
- Identify and mark tender area at mid-point of tendon
- Insert needle horizontally at the lateral edge of the patellar tendon just proximal to the tibial tubercle. Ensure that the needle does not enter the tendon
- Deposit solution as bolus

Aftercare The patient must avoid all overuse of the knee for at least 1 week. When the cause is occupational, such as in carpet layers, a pad with a hole in it to relieve pressure on the bursa should be used.

Graded stretching and strengthening exercises are then begun.

Comments It would be tempting to believe that pain found at mid-point of the patella tendon is caused by tendinitis, but in the experience of the authors this is virtually unknown. Infrapatellar tendinitis is found consistently at the proximal teno-osseous junction on the patella, or rarely at insertion into the tibial tubercle. Pain here in an adolescent boy should be considered to be Osgood Schlatter's disease and should not be injected.

A similar approach can be used for the superficial bursa and for the prepatellar bursa.

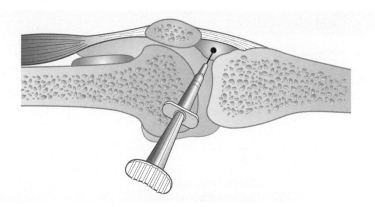

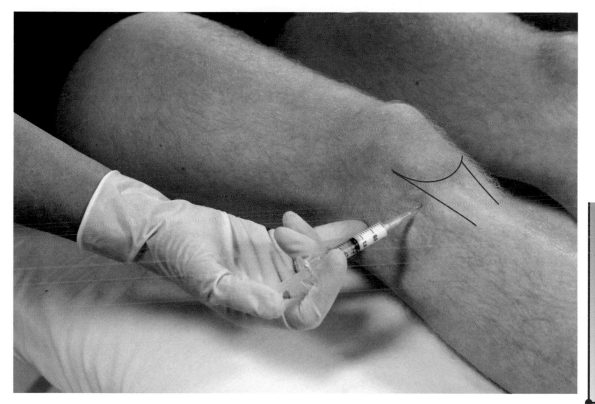

PES ANSEURINE BURSA

Chronic bursitis

Causes and findings
- Overuse – especially dancers or runners
- Pain just proximal to insertion of medial flexors of knee
- Painful: resisted flexion of knee

Equipment

Syringe	Needle	Kenalog 40	Lidocaine	Total volume
2 ml	23G 1.25 inches (30 mm) Blue	20 mg	1.5 ml 2%	2 ml

Anatomy
The pes anseurine is the combined tendon of insertion of the sartorius, gracilis and semi-tendinosus. It attaches on the medial side of the tibia just below the knee joint line. The bursa lies immediately under the tendon just posterior to its insertion and is extremely tender to palpation in the normal knee.

Technique
- Patient sits with knee supported
- Identify the pes anseurine tendon by making patient strongly flex knee against resistance. Follow the combined tendons distally to where they disappear at insertion into tibia. The bursa is found as an area of extreme tenderness slightly proximal to the insertion
- Insert needle into centre of tender area through tendon until it touches bone
- Deposit solution in bolus

Aftercare
The patient should avoid overuse activities for at least 1 week, when graded stretching and strengthening exercises are started.

Comments
It is important to remember that the bursa is extremely tender to palpation on everybody, so comparison testing must be done on both knees.

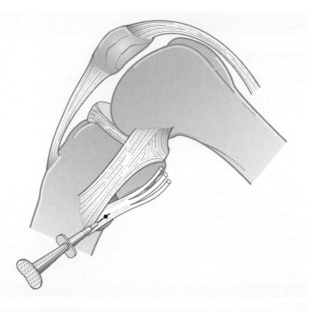

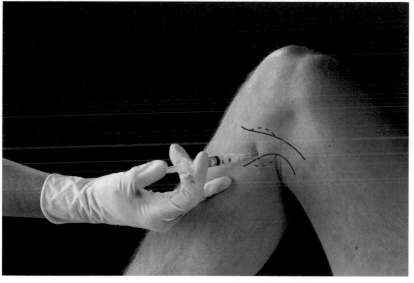

ILIOTIBIAL BAND BURSA

Chronic bursitis

Causes and findings
- Overuse – especially long-distance runners
- Pain on the outer side of the knee above the lateral femoral condyle
- Painful:
  resisted abduction of leg
  passive adduction of leg

Equipment

Syringe	Needle	Kenalog 40	Lidocaine	Total volume
2 ml	23G 1 inch (25 mm) Blue	20 mg	1.5 ml 2%	2 ml

Anatomy
The bursa lies deep to the iliotibial band just above the lateral condyle of the femur.

Technique
- Patient sits with knee supported
- Identify and mark tender area on lateral side of femur
- Insert needle into bursa passing through tendon to touch bone
- Deposit solution in bolus

Aftercare
Absolute rest must be maintained for about 10 days and then a stretching and strengthening programme initiated.
Footwear and running technique should be checked and corrected if necessary.

Comments
The lower end of the iliotibial tract itself can be irritated, but invariably the bursa is also at fault. If both lesions are suspected, infiltration of both at the same time can be performed.

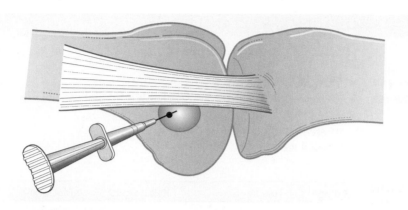

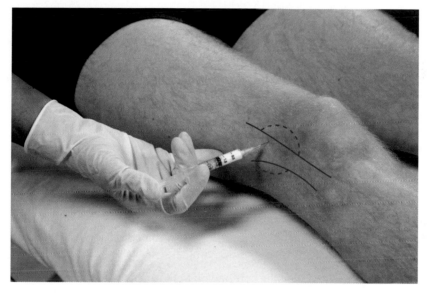

QUADRICEPS EXPANSION

Muscle sprain

Causes and findings
- Overuse
- Pain usually on superior medial side of patella
- Painful:
  on going down hill or down stairs
  resisted extension of the knee

Equipment

Syringe	Needle	Kenalog 40	Lidocaine	Total volume
2 ml	25G 0.5 inch (16 mm) Orange	10 mg	1.75 ml 2%	2 ml

Anatomy The quadriceps muscle inserts as an expansion around the borders of the patella. The usual site of the lesion is at the superior medial pole of the patella. This is found by pushing the patella medially with the thumb and palpating up and under the medial edge with a finger to find the tender area.

Technique
- Patient half lies on table with knee relaxed
- Identify and mark tender area usually on medial edge of superior pole of patella
- Insert needle and angle horizontally to touch bone of patella
- Pepper solution along line of insertion

Aftercare Patient avoids overusing the knee for at least 1 week and, when pain free, begins progressive strengthening and stretching programme.

Comments This lesion, like the coronary ligament, responds very well to two or three sessions of strong deep friction. The injection is used therefore when the friction is not available, the area is too tender, or to disinflame the expansion prior to friction a week later, in a combination approach. The same technique may be used to inject inflamed plicae around the patella rim.

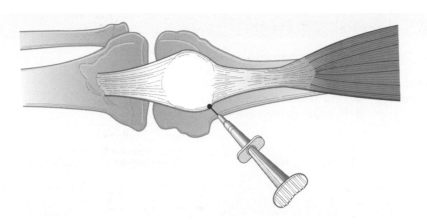

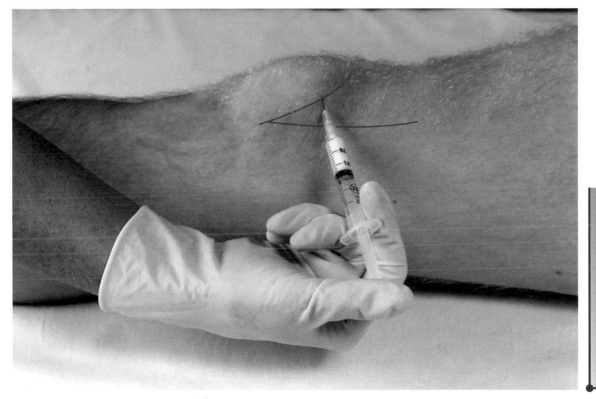

INFRAPATELLAR TENDON

Chronic tendinitis

Causes and findings
- Overuse – jumpers and runners
- Pain at inferior pole of patella
- Painful: resisted extension of knee

Equipment

Syringe	Needle	Kenalog 40	Lidocaine	Total volume
2 ml	23G 1.25 inches (30 mm) Blue	20 mg	1.5 ml 2%	2 ml

Anatomy
The infrapatellar tendon arises from the inferior pole of the patella and it is here that it is commonly inflamed. The tendon is at least two fingers wide at its origin.

It is an absolute contraindication to inject corticosteroid into the body of the tendon as it is a large, weight-bearing and relatively avascular structure. Tenderness at mid-point of the tendon is usually caused by infrapatellar bursitis.

Technique
- Patient sits with knee supported and extended
- Place web of cephalic hand on superior pole of patella and tilt inferior pole up. Identify and mark tender area at origin of tendon on distal end of patella
- Insert needle at mid-point of tendon origin at an angle of 45°
- Pepper solution along tendon in two rows. There should always be some resistance to the needle to ensure that the solution is not being introduced intra-articularly

Aftercare
Absolute rest is recommended for at least 10 days before a stretching and strengthening programme is initiated.

Comments
Injecting the origin of the infrapatellar tendon at the inferior pole is very safe, provided adequate rest is maintained afterwards and that no more than two injections are given in one attack. In an ageing patient with a chronic tendinopathy, scanning is recommended first to ensure that there are no degenerative changes in the substance of the tendon.

Alternative approach
In the case of the committed athlete or if scanning shows changes as above, deep friction, electrotherapy and taping should be given as potential danger of rupture is more real.

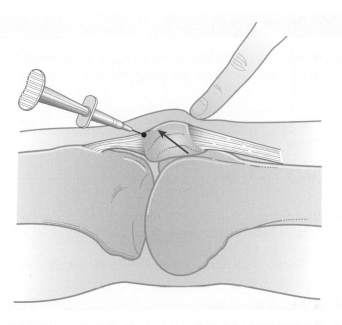

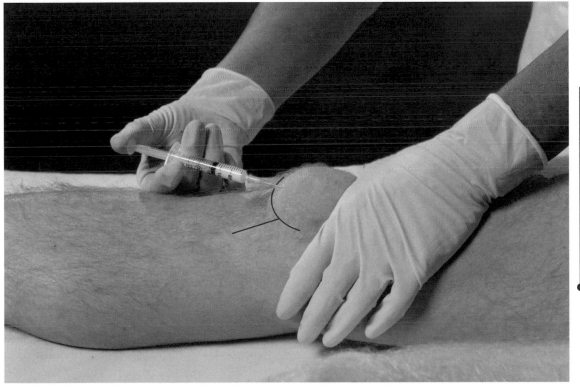

BAKER'S CYST

Causes and findings
- Spontaneous insidious onset, usually in osteoarthritic joint
- Obvious swelling in the popliteal fossa – often quite large

Equipment

Syringe	Needle	Kenalog 40	Lidocaine	Total volume
10 ml	19G 1.5 inches (40 mm) Green			

Anatomy
Baker's cyst is a sac of synovial fluid caused by seepage through a defect in the posterior wall of the capsule of the knee joint, or by effusion within the semi-membranosus bursa.

The popliteal artery and vein and posterior tibial nerve pass centrally in the popliteal fossa and must be avoided.

Technique
- Patient lies prone
- Mark spot two fingers medial to mid-line of fossa and two fingers below the popliteal crease
- Insert needle at marked spot and angle laterally at 45° angle
- Aspirate fluid found

Aftercare
A firm compression bandage can be applied for a day or two.

Comments
If anything other than clear synovial fluid is removed, a specimen should be sent for culture and the appropriate treatment instigated. Invariably the swelling returns at some point but can be re-aspirated if the patient wishes.

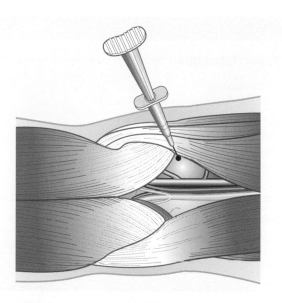

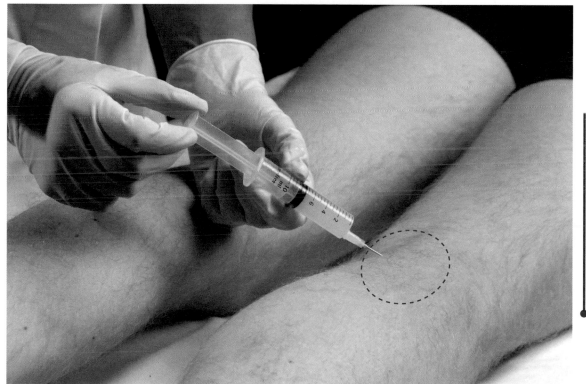

ANKLE JOINT

Chronic capsulitis

Causes and findings
- Post-trauma
- Pain at front of, or within, ankle
- Painful and limited:
  more passive plantarflexion
  less passive dorsiflexion

Equipment

Syringe	Needle	Kenalog 40	Lidocaine	Total volume
2 ml	23G 1.25 inches (30 mm) Blue	30 mg	1.25 ml 2%	2 ml

Anatomy
The easiest and safest entry point to the ankle joint is at the junction of the tibia and fibula just above the talus. A small triangular space can be palpated there.

Technique
- Patient lies with knee bent to 90° and foot slightly plantarflexed
- Identify and mark small triangular space by passively flexing and extending the ankle while palpating
- Insert needle into joint angling slightly medially and proximally to pass into joint space
- Deposit solution as bolus

Aftercare
Excessive weight-bearing activities are avoided for at least 1 week. The patient should be warned that heavy overuse of the foot will cause a recurrence of symptoms and therefore long-distance running should be avoided. Weight control is also advised and footwear should be checked to ensure correct support.

Comments
The ankle joint rarely causes problems except after severe trauma or fracture, and then often many years later. The infiltration is usually very successful in giving long-lasting pain relief and can be repeated if necessary at intervals of at least 3 months with an annual X-ray to monitor degenerative changes.

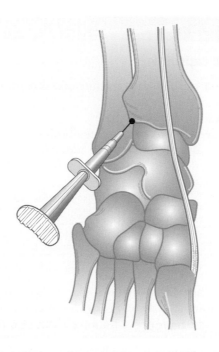

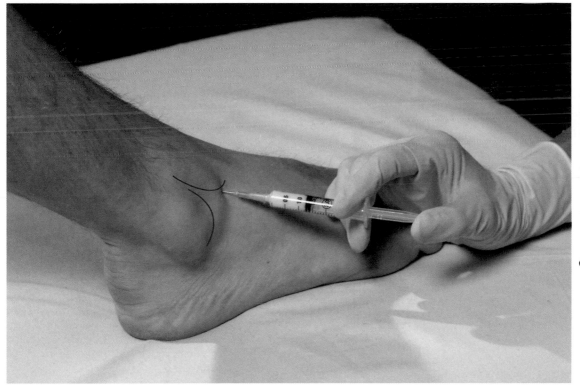

SUBTALAR JOINT

Chronic capsulitis

Causes and findings
- Trauma – usually after fracture or severe impaction injury, often many years later
- Overuse in the older obese
- Pain deep in medial and lateral sides of heel
- Painful and limited: passive adduction of the calcaneus

Equipment

Syringe	Needle	Kenalog 40	Lidocaine	Total volume
2 ml	23G 1.25 inches (30 mm) Blue	30 mg	1.25 ml 2%	2 ml

Anatomy
The subtalar joint is divided by an oblique septum into anterior and posterior portions. It is slightly easier to enter the joint just above the sustentaculum tali, which projects a thumb's width directly below the medial malleolus.

Technique
- Patient lies on side with foot supported so that medial aspect of heel faces upwards
- Identify bump of sustentaculum tali
- Insert needle perpendicularly immediately above and slightly posterior to sustentaculum tali
- Deposit half solution here
- Withdraw needle slightly and angle obliquely anteriorly through septum into anterior compartment of joint space and deposit remaining solution here

Aftercare
The patient should avoid excessive weight-bearing activities for at least 1 week. Orthotics and weight control are helpful in preventing recurrence.

Comments
This is a difficult injection to perform due to the anatomical shape of the joint. It can be repeated at infrequent intervals if necessary.

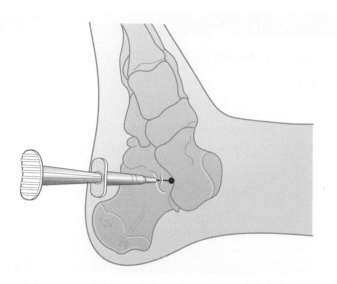

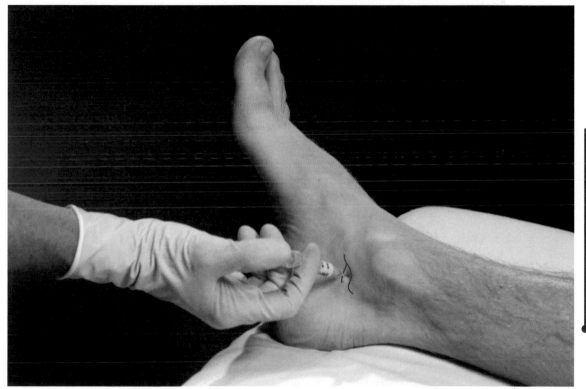

DELTOID LIGAMENT

Acute or chronic sprain

Causes and findings
- Trauma
- Obesity
- Overpronation of the foot
- Pain over medial side of heel below medial malleolus
- Painful: passive eversion of ankle in plantarflexion

Equipment

Syringe	Needle	Kenalog 40	Lidocaine	Total volume
1 ml	25G 0.5 inch (16mm) Orange	10mg	0.75 ml 2%	1 ml

Anatomy
The deltoid ligament is a strong cuboid structure with two layers. It runs from the medial malleolus to the sustentaculum tali on the calcaneum and to the tubercle on the navicular. Sprains here are not as common as at the lateral ligament, but because they do not seem to respond well to friction and mobilization, injection is worth trying. The inflamed part is usually at the origin on the malleolus.

Technique
- Patient sits with medial side of foot accessible
- Identify lower border of medial malleolus and mark mid-point of ligament
- Insert needle and angle upwards to touch bone at mid-point of ligament
- Pepper solution along attachment to bone

Aftercare
Activity should be limited for at least 1 week. To prevent recurrence, the bio-mechanics of the foot must be carefully checked. Orthotics are almost always necessary and, in the overweight patient, advice on diet must be given.

Comments
This is an uncommon but usually successful injection.

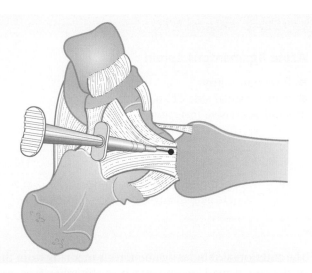

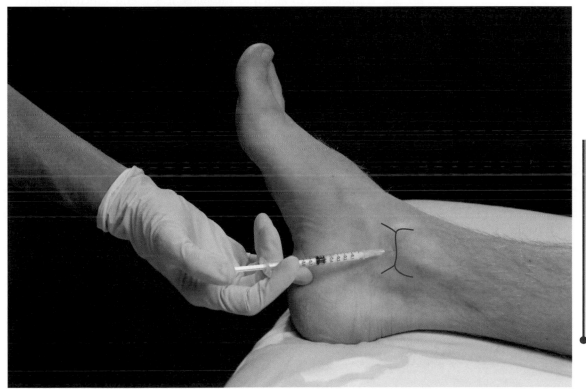

LATERAL LIGAMENT

Acute ligamentous sprain

Causes and findings
- Inversion injury
- Pain at lateral side of ankle
- Painful: passive inversion of ankle

Equipment

Syringe	Needle	Kenalog 40	Lidocaine	Total volume
1 ml	25G 0.5 inch (16 mm) Orange	10 mg	0.75 ml 2%	1 ml

Anatomy
The anterior talofibular ligament runs medially from the anterior inferior edge of the lateral malleolus to attach to the talus. It is a thin structure, approximately the width of the little finger.

The bifurcate calcaneocuboid ligament runs from the calcaneus to the cuboid and is often also involved in ankle sprains. Both ligaments run parallel to the sole of the foot.

Technique
- Patient lies supported on table
- Identify and mark anterior inferior edge of lateral malleolus
- Insert needle to touch bone
- Pepper half solution around origin of ligament
- Turn needle and pepper remainder into insertion on talus

Aftercare
Patient keeps ankle moving within pain-free range. For the first few days, ice, elevation and taping in eversion are helpful, together with a pressure pad behind the malelleous to control swelling. Exercises to strengthen the peronei and proprioception usually need to be given.

Comments
This injection is an option when the pain is very acute or where conservative treatment has failed in the chronic stage.

Alternative approaches
This lesion responds very well in the acute stage to a regime of ice, elevation, gentle massage, active and passive mobilization and taping.

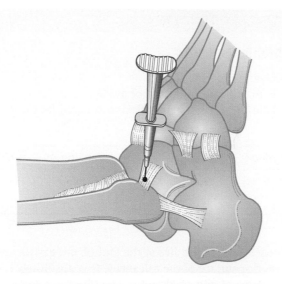

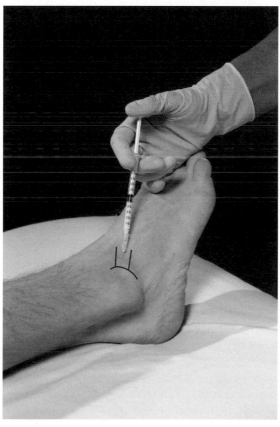

ACHILLES TENDON

Chronic tendinitis

Causes and findings
- Overuse
- Pain at posterior aspect of ankle
- Painful: resisted plantarflexion on one foot or from full dorsiflexion

Equipment

Syringe	Needle	Kenalog 40	Lidocaine	Total volume
2 ml	23G 1.25 inches (30 mm) Blue	20 mg	1.5 ml 2%	2 ml

Anatomy
The achilles tendon lies at the end of the gastrocnemius as it inserts into the posterior surface of the calcaneus. It is absolutely contraindicated to infiltrate the body of the tendon because this is a large, weight-bearing, relatively avascular tendon with a known propensity to rupture.

Technique
- Patient lies prone with foot held in dorsiflexion over end of bed. This keeps the tendon under tension and facilitates the procedure
- Identify and mark tender area of tendon – usually along the sides
- Insert needle on medial side and angle parallel to tendon. Slide needle along side of tendon, taking care not to enter into tendon itself
- Deposit half solution while slowly withdrawing needle
- Insert needle on lateral side and repeat procedure with remaining half of solution

Aftercare
Absolute avoidance of any overuse is essential for about 10 days. Deep friction to the site should then be given a few times, even if the patient is asymptomatic, to prevent recurrence. When pain free, graded stretching and strengthening exercises are begun and should be continued indefinitely. Orthotics and retraining in the causal activity are often necessary.

Comments
Although there are reports of tendon rupture after injection here, this has usually occurred as a result of repeated injections of large dose and volume into the body of a degenerate tendon and with excessive exercise post-injection. Because of this recognized risk therefore, we recommend scanning the tendon prior to injecting to ascertain the extent of the degeneration (Chapter 2). Clear degenerative changes within the substance, rather than just around the periphery, would indicate an absolute contraindication to injection.

Depositing the solution along the sides is safe and effective but should not be repeated more than once in one attack. The committed athlete should preferably be offered deep friction and a graduated stretching/strengthening programme.

Alternative approaches
No one method has been entirely successful in treating this condition. Recent novel approaches include the continuous application of topical glyceryl trinitrate and injection of a sclerosing local anaesthetic (Polidocanol; see Chapter 1).

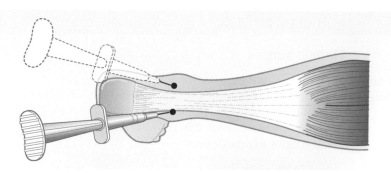

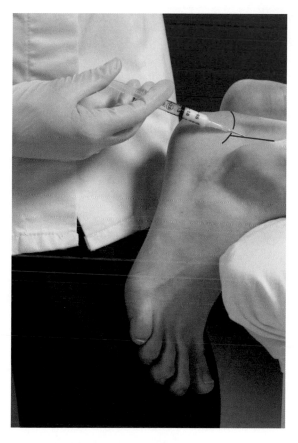

ACHILLES BURSA

Chronic bursitis

Causes and findings
- Overuse – runners and dancers
- Pain posterior to tibia and anterior to body of Achilles tendon
- Painful:
  resisted plantarflexion, especially at end range
  full passive plantarflexion

Equipment

Syringe	Needle	Kenalog 40	Lidocaine	Total volume
2 ml	23G 1.25 inches (30 mm) Blue	20 mg	1.5 ml 2%	2 ml

Anatomy
The Achilles bursa lies in the triangular space anterior to the tendon and posterior to the base of the tibia and the upper part of the calcaneus.

It is important to differentiate between tendinitis and bursitis here because both are caused by overuse. In bursitis there is usually more pain on full passive plantarflexion when the heel is pressed up against the back of the tibia, thereby squeezing the bursa. Also, palpation of the bursa is very sensitive and the pain is usually felt more at the end of rising on tip-toe rather than during the movement.

The best approach is from the lateral side to avoid the posterior tibial artery and nerve.

Technique
- Patient lies prone with foot held in some dorsiflexion
- Identify and mark tender area on lateral side of bursa
- Insert needle into bursa avoiding piercing the tendon
- Deposit solution as bolus

Aftercare
Avoid overuse activities for at least 10 days, then start a stretching and eccentric exercise programme. Female ballet dancers need to avoid over-plantarflexing the ankle when on point.

Comments
It is important to avoid penetrating the Achilles tendon and depositing the solution there. Any resistance to the needle requires immediate withdrawal and repositioning well anterior to the tendon.

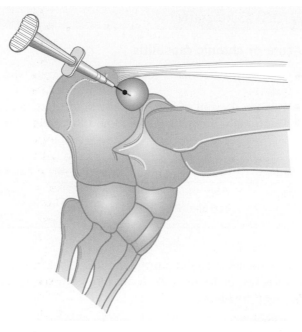

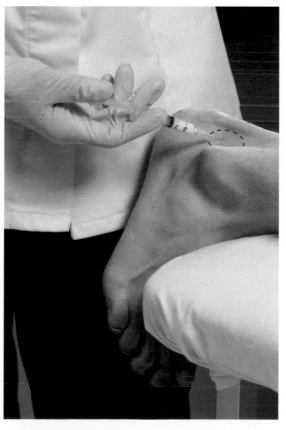

MIDTARSAL JOINTS

Acute or chronic capsulitis

Causes and findings
- Overuse or trauma – female ballet dancers who over-point or football players
- Pain on dorsum of foot – usually at third metatarsocuneiform joint line
- Painful and limited: adduction and inversion of midtarsal joints

Equipment

Syringe	Needle	Kenalog 40	Lidocaine	Total volume
2 ml	23G 1 inch (25 mm) Blue	20 mg	1.5 ml 2%	2 ml

Anatomy
There are several joints in the mid-tarsus, each with its own capsule. Gross passive testing followed by local joint gliding and palpation should identify the joint involved.

Technique
- Patient lies with foot supported in neutral
- Identify and mark tender joint line
- Insert needle down into joint space
- Pepper some solution into capsule and remainder as bolus into joint cavity

Aftercare
Avoidance of excessive weight-bearing activities for at least 1 week is advised. Mobilizing and strengthening exercises and retraining of causal activities follow. Orthotics and weight control, if necessary, are useful additions.

Comments
This is a successful treatment provided sensible attention is paid to aftercare.

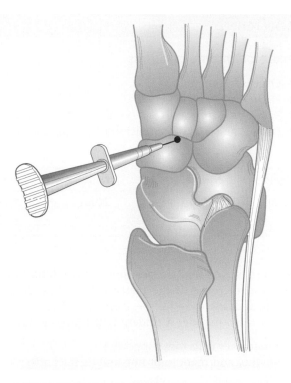

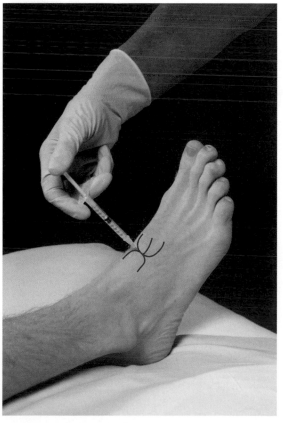

TOE JOINTS

Acute or chronic capsulitis

Causes and findings
- Overuse or trauma
- Hallux valgus
- Pain in toe joint
- Painful and limited: extension of the big toe, flexion of other toes

Equipment

Syringe	Needle	Kenalog 40	Lidocaine	Total volume
2 ml	25G 0.5 inch (16 mm) Orange	20 mg	1 ml 2%	1.5 ml

Anatomy
The first metatarsophalangeal joint line is found by palpating the space produced at the base of the metacarpal on the dorsal aspect, while passively flexing and extending the toe. Palpation of the collateral ligaments at the joint line of the other toes will identify the affected joint or joints.

Technique
- Patient lies with foot supported
- Identify and mark joint line and distract affected toe with one hand
- Insert needle perpendicularly into joint space avoiding extensor tendons
- Deposit solution as bolus

Aftercare
Avoidance of excessive weight-bearing activities for at least 1 week, together with taping of the joint and a toe pad between the toes. Care in choice of footwear and orthotics might be necessary.

Comments
As with the thumb joint injection, this treatment can be very long-lasting.

The other toe joints are injected from the medial or lateral aspect while under traction.

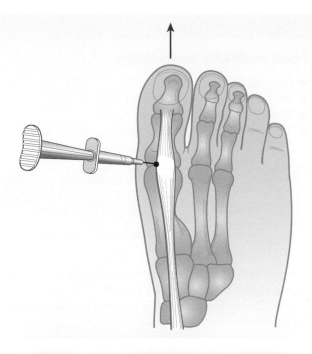

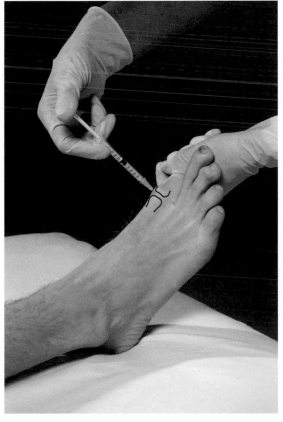

PERONEAL TENDONS

Acute or chronic tendinopathy

Causes and findings
- Overuse
- Pain at lateral side of ankle or foot
- Painful: resisted eversion of the foot
- Tender area above, behind or below the lateral malleolus

Equipment

Syringe	Needle	Kenalog 40	Lidocaine	Total volume
1 ml	25G 0.5 inch (16 mm) Orange	10 mg	0.75 ml 2%	1 ml

Anatomy
The peroneus longus and brevis run together in a synovial sheath behind the lateral malleolus. The longus then divides to pass under the arch of the foot to insert at the base of the big toe, and brevis inserts into the base of the fifth metatarsal.

The division of the two tendons is the entry point for the needle and can be found by having the patient hold the foot in strong eversion and palpating for the V-shaped fork of the tendons.

Technique
- Patient lies supine with foot supported in some medial rotation
- Identify and mark division of the two tendons
- Insert needle perpendicularly at this point, turn and slide horizontally under skin towards malleolus
- Deposit solution into combined tendon sheath. There should be minimal resistance and often a sausage-shaped bulge is observed

Aftercare
Avoid any overuse for about 1 week. Resolution of symptoms should then lead to consideration of change in footwear, orthotics and strengthening of the evertors.

Comments
Occasionally the tendinopathy occurs at the insertion of the peroneus brevis. The same amount of solution is then peppered into the teno-osseous junction by inserting the needle parallel to the skin to touch the base of the fifth metatarsal.

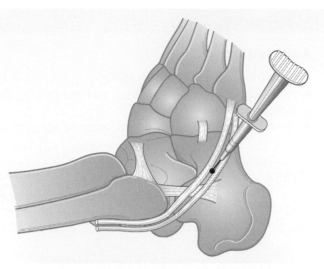

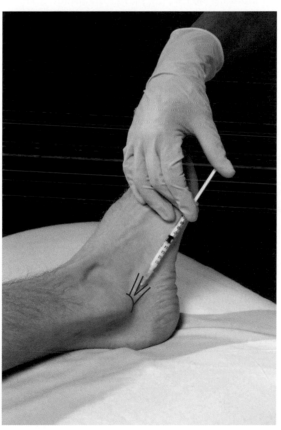

PLANTAR FASCIA

Acute fasciitis

Causes and findings
- Idiopathic, overuse, poor footwear
- Pain on medial aspect of heel pad on putting foot to ground in the morning
- Tender area over medial edge of origin of fascia from calcaneus

Equipment

Syringe	Needle	Kenalog 40	Lidocaine	Total volume
2 ml	21G 1.5–2 inches (40–50 mm) Green	20 mg	1.5 ml 2%	2 ml

Anatomy
The plantar fascia, or long plantar ligament, arises from the medial and lateral tubercles on the inferior surface of the calcaneus. The lesion is always found at the medial head and the area of irritation can be palpated by deep pressure with the thumb.

Technique
- Patient lies prone with foot supported in dorsiflexion
- Identify tender area on heel
- Insert needle perpendicularly into medial side of soft part of sole just distal to heel pad. Advance at 45° towards calcaneus until it touches bone
- Pepper solution in two rows into fascia at its medial bony origin

Aftercare
A heel support is used for at least 1 week after the injection, followed by intrinsic muscle exercise and stretching of the fascia. Standing on a golf ball to apply deep friction can be helpful and orthotics can be applied. Taping can also be used.

Comments
Although this would appear to be an extremely painful injection, this approach is much kinder than inserting the needle straight through the heel pad, and patients tolerate it well.

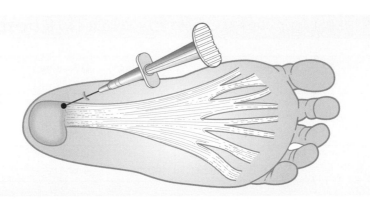

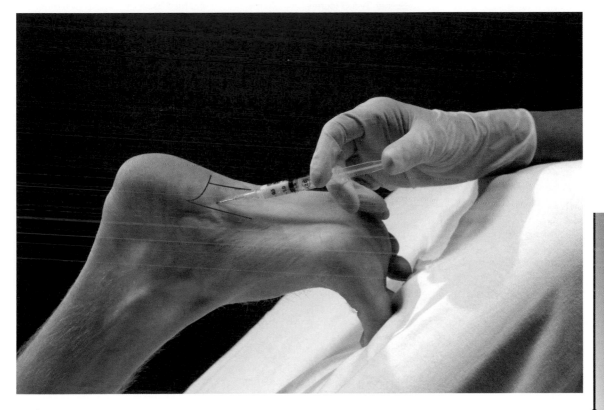

SUMMARY OF SUGGESTED LOWER LIMB DOSES

Syringe	Needle	Kenalog 40	Lidocaine	Total volume
Hip				
Hip joint 5 ml	Spinal 3–3.5 inches	40 mg	4 ml 1%	5 ml
Gluteal bursa 5 ml	Spinal 3–3.5 inches	40 mg	4 ml 1%	5 ml
Psoas bursa 5 ml	Spinal 3–3.5 inches	20 mg	4.5 ml 1%	5 ml
Trochanteric bursa 2 ml	Blue 1.25 inches	20 mg	1.5 ml 2%	2 ml
Adductor tendon 2 ml	Blue 1.25 inches	20 mg	1.5 ml 2%	2 ml
Hamstring tendon/bursitis 2 ml	Green 1.5–2 inches	20 mg	1.5 ml 2%	2 ml
Lateral cutaneous nerve 1 ml	Green 2 inches	20 mg	Nil	0.5 ml
Knee				
Knee joint 5–10 ml	Green 1.5 inches	40 mg	4 ml 1%–9 ml 0.5%	5–10 ml
Superior tibiofibular joint 2 ml	Blue 1 inch	20 mg	1 ml 2%	1.5 ml
Coronary ligament 1 ml	Orange 0.5 inch	10 mg	0.75 ml 2%	1 ml
Medial collateral ligament 2 ml	Blue 1.25 inches	20 mg	1 ml 2%	1.5 ml
Infrapatellar bursa 2 ml	Blue 1.25 inches	20 mg	1.5 ml 2%	2 ml
Pes anseurine bursa 2 ml	Blue 1.25 inches	20 mg	1.5 ml 2%	2 ml
Iliotibial bursa 2 ml	Blue 1 inch	20 mg	1.5 ml 2%	2 ml
Quadriceps expansion 1 ml	Orange 0.5 inch	10 mg	1.75 ml 2%	2 ml
Infrapatellar tendon 2 ml	Blue 1.25 inches	20 mg	1.5 ml 2%	2 ml
Ankle and foot				
Ankle joint 2 ml	Blue 1.25 inches	30 mg	1.25 ml 2%	2 ml
Subtalar joint 2 ml	Blue 1.25 inches	30 mg	1.25 ml 2%	2 ml

Syringe	Needle	Kenalog 40	Lidocaine	Total volume
Deltoid ligament 1 ml	Orange 0.5 inch	10 mg	0.75 ml 2%	1 ml
Lateral ligament 1 ml	Orange 0.5 inch	10 mg	0.75 ml 2%	1 ml
Achilles tendon 2 ml	Blue 1.25 inches	20 mg	1.5 ml 2%	2 ml
Achilles bursa 2 ml	Blue 1.25 inches	20 mg	1.5 ml 2%	2 ml
Midtarsal joints 2 ml	Blue 1 inch	20 mg	1.5 ml 2%	2 ml
Big toe/toe joints 2 ml	Orange 0.5 inch	20 mg	1 ml 2%	1.5 ml
Peroneal tendons 1 ml	Orange 0.5 inch	10 mg	0.75 ml 2%	1 ml
Plantar fascia 2 ml	Green 1.5–2 inches	20 mg	1.5 ml 2%	2 ml

INJECTION TECHNIQUES: SPINE AND JAW

Finger measurements are from the patient, not the clinician.

SPINAL INJECTIONS

INTRODUCTION There is some controversy in the literature regarding spinal injections[98,99,127–134,151–154,231,315]. Depot steroids are not licensed for spinal use[135,136] but orthopaedic and pain specialists, rheumatologists and others use these injections extensively[258] (see the section Use of drugs beyond licence, p 23). There is currently no consensus about epidural injection techniques and wide variations in current practice[150].

A Cochrane systematic review recommends that because of the tendency towards positive results favouring injection therapy, and the minor side-effects reported by the reviewed studies, there is at the moment no justification for abandoning this treatment for patients with low back pain. However, because of the lack of statistically significant results, as well as the lack of well-designed trials, a solid foundation for the effectiveness of injection therapy is also lacking[133].

ACCURACY Corticosteroids, often mixed with a local anaesthetic, can be injected into the epidural space (via the caudal or lumbar route), around nerve roots, into or around the facet and sacroiliac joints and into muscle trigger points. Performing the injection under fluoroscopy can ensure correct placement of spinal injections[137,139] but many doctors perform these techniques 'blind' and obtain satisfactory results.[289] The accuracy of blind caudal epidural injections has been assessed in two studies. In one, successful injection placement on the first attempt occurred in three out of four subjects. Results were improved when anatomical landmarks were identified easily (88%) and no air was palpable subcutaneously over the sacrum when injected through the needle (83%). The combination of these two signs predicted a successful injection in 91% of attempts[289]. In the other study blind injections were correctly placed in only two out of three attempts, even when the operator was confident of accurate placement. When the operator was less certain, the success rate was less than half. If the patient was obese the success rate reduced even further[137].

VOLUME In the past, large volumes have been injected into the epidural space[138], however, a total injection volume of 8 ml is sufficient for a caudal epidural injection to reach the L4/5 level[139].

EFFICACY The number needed to treat (NNT) with epidural corticosteroids for greater than 75% pain relief in the short term (1–60 days) is 7 (confidence interval = 5–16). The NNT for greater than 50% pain relief in the long term (3–12 months) is 13 (CI = 7–314)[99].

Selective nerve-root injections of corticosteroids (under X-ray control) are significantly more effective than those of bupivacaine alone in obviating the

SECTION 4

need for operative decompression for 13–28 months following the injections in operative candidates. This finding suggests that patients who have lumbar radicular pain at one or two levels should be considered for treatment with selective nerve-root injections of corticosteroids prior to operative intervention[132]. When symptoms have been present for more than 12 months, local anaesthetic alone may be just as effective as steroid and local anaesthetic together[257].

Injection of the sacroiliac joints for painful sacroiliitis appears to be safe and effective. It can be considered in patients with contraindications or complications with NSAIDs, or if other medical treatment is ineffective[210].

When conservative measures fail, nerve-root injections are effective in reducing radicular pain in patients with osteoporotic vertebral fractures and no evidence of nerve root palsy. These patients may be considered for this treatment before percutaneous vertebroplasty or operative intervention is attempted[234].

SCLEROSANTS

Sclerosant injections are used to treat back pain with presumed ligamentous insufficiency[140,230,232,291]. They may be ineffective in patients with very long-standing (e.g. 10 years) back pain and features of psychosocial distress[141], and are not shown here.

SAFETY

The incidence of intravascular uptake during lumbar spinal injection procedures is approximately 8.5%. It is greater in patients over 50, and if the caudal route is used rises to 11%. Absence of flashback of blood on preinjection aspiration does not predict extravascular needle placement[288]. Epidural steroid injection is safe in patients receiving aspirin-like antiplatelet medications, with no excess risk of serious haemorrhagic complications, i.e. spinal haematoma. Increased age, needle gauge, needle approach, needle insertion at multiple interspaces, number of needle passes, volume of injectant and accidental dural puncture are risk factors for minor haemorrhagic complications. New neurological symptoms or worsening of pre-existing complaints that persist for more than 24 hours (median duration of symptoms 3 days, range 1–20 days) might occur after epidural injection[163].

Anticoagulant therapy with warfarin is an absolute contraindication to spinal injection.

Safety precautions and strict aseptic techniques are the same as for all injections but an additional hazard is the rare possibility of an intrathecal injection of local anaesthetic. For this reason some practitioners use corticosteroid alone, without the addition of anaesthetic. The rationale is that the benefit of the brief relief of pain and the diagnostic information obtained from using anaesthetic does not outweigh the potential risks. Normal saline can be added if additional volume is required.

The British Society for Rheumatology (2001) and the Royal College of Anaesthetists (2002) have produced guidelines for the use of epidural injections. We commend them to all practitioners who give these injections. They can be found at:

- www.rheumatology.org.uk
- www.rcoa.ac.uk

For physicians using this guide, there follows a description of spinal injections that can be carried out safely in an outpatient setting provided resuscitation facilities are available and appropriate guidelines are strictly followed. We strongly recommend that doctors attend recognized training courses and undergo a period of supervised practice with an experienced colleague before attempting them on their own. Revisiting the anatomy laboratory before perfoming any spinal injections is an essential part of the training process.

ASSESSMENT OF THE SPINE

Cervical spine tests

Active: flexion
             rotations
             side flexions
             extension

Passive: rotations
             side flexions
             extension

Resisted: shoulder abduction C5
             shoulder lateral rotation C5
             shoulder medial rotation C6
             elbow flexion C6
             elbow extension C7
             shoulder adduction C7
             wrist extension C6
             wrist flexion C7
             thumb extension C8
             finger adduction T1

Reflexes: brachioradialis C5, biceps C6, triceps C7

Cervical capsular pattern: equal loss of rotations and side flexions, more loss of extension than flexion

---

Lumbar spine tests

Active: extension
             side flexions
             flexion

Passive: hip flexion
             hip rotations

             straight leg raise

Resisted: foot plantarflexion S1
             hip flexion L2
             foot dorsiflexion L4
             big toe extension L4/5

Resisted: foot eversion L5/S1
             knee extension L3
             knee flexion S1
             glutei S1

Reflexes: knee L3, ankle L5, S1/2

Lumbar capsular pattern: equal loss of side flexions, more loss of extension than flexion

CERVICAL FACET JOINTS

Acute or chronic capsulitis

Causes and findings
- Osteoarthritis, rheumatoid arthritis or traumatic capsulitis
- Pain in posterior neck, up to head, into scapula or to point of shoulder
- Increased by sleeping in awkward positions and end-of-range movement
- Painful limitation in the capsular pattern: both rotations, side flexions and extension
- Tender over one or more facet joints

Equipment

Syringe	Needle	Kenalog 40	Lidocaine	Total volume
1 ml	21G 1.5–2 inches (40–50 mm) Green	20 mg	Nil	0.5 ml

Anatomy
The facet or zygaphophyseal joints in the cervical spine are plane joints lying at angles of approximately 30–45° to the vertical. They can be palpated by identifying the spinous process and moving a finger's width laterally, and are felt as a flat pillar. The affected levels are sensitive to pressure.

Technique
- Patient lies on unaffected side with roll under neck
- Neck is held in flexion and slight side flexion away from the painful side
- Identify and mark the tender joint
- Insert needle just distal to joint parallel to the spinous processes and angle upwards at an angle of 45° cephalad
- Pass through the thick extensors aiming towards patient's upper ear until point touches bone
- Aspirate to ensure needle point is not intrathecal
- Gently 'walk' along bone until needle touches joint capsule – a hard end-feel
- Inject solution in bolus intracapsular or pepper into capsule

Aftercare
Patient maintains gentle movement, continues correct posture and is careful to sleep with a suitable number of pillows to maintain the head in a neutral position. Prone lying should be abandoned. Manual traction, mobilizing and sustained stretching techniques together with friction massage to the joint capsule helps maintain comfortable movement.

Comments
Although this appears to be an alarming injection, it is perfectly safe provided great care is taken that the needle always lies parallel to the spinous process and never angles medially, and that the point touches bone before depositing the solution. The results in the osteoarthritic neck can be good for several months, provided the patient does not strain the neck and maintains mobility and good posture as above.

Alternative approach
This injection can be done under imaging which ensures correct placement but is less cost effective.

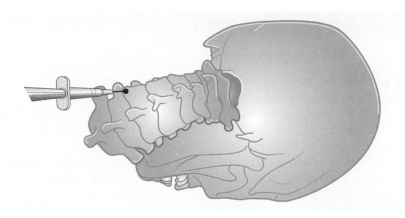

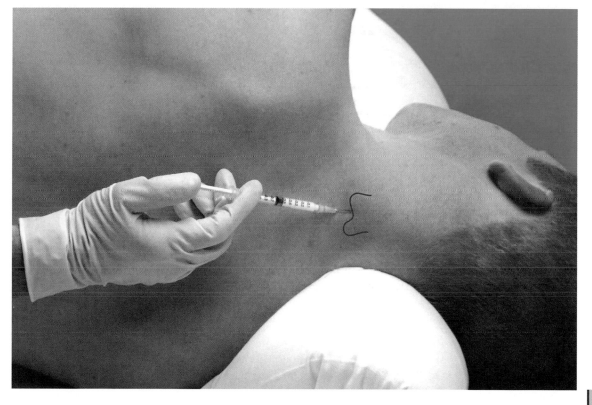

LUMBAR FACET JOINTS

Chronic capsulitis

Causes and findings
- Osteoarthritis or traumatic capsulitis, ankylosing spondylitis
- Spondylolysis/spondylolysthesis
- Unilateral low back pain, sometimes with dull vague aching down leg
- Painful limitation in the capsular pattern – most: loss of extension; less: loss of both side flexions; least: loss of flexion
- In younger patients with spondylolysis, often most painful movement is combined extension with side flexion to the painful side

Equipment

Syringe	Needle	Kenalog 40	Lidocaine	Total volume
1 ml	22G 3–3.5 inches (75–90 mm) Spinal	40 mg	Nil	1 ml

Anatomy
The lower lumbar facet or zygaphophyseal joints lie lateral to the spinous processes – approximately one finger width at L3, one and a half at L4 and two fingers' width at L5. They cannot be palpated but are located by marking a vertical line along the centre of the spinous processes and horizontal lines across *between* each process. The posterior capsule of the joint is found by inserting the needle the correct distance for that level laterally on the horizontal line.

Technique
- Patient lies prone on small pillow to aid localization of the spinous interspace
- Identify and mark one or more tender levels
- Insert needle at first selected level vertically down to capsule
- Aspirate to ensure needle point is not intrathecal
- Deposit solution into and around capsule
- Withdraw needle and repeat at different levels if necessary

Aftercare
Patient avoids excessive movement while maintaining activity. Abdominal strengthening and mobilizing exercises should be performed regularly. Occasional mobilization and hamstring stretching will help to maintain flexibility.

Comments
If the capsule is not found immediately, gently 'walk' needle around bone until a hard end-feel is reached.

Alternative approach
Some practitioners perform injection of the lumbar facets under fluoroscopy, but they can be safely reached in the above manner provided the end-point of the needle on bone is reached. This approach is more cost effective.

Transforaminal Nerve Block

> Versed - 2 mgs.

1 ml. Kenalog 40 mg - Fentanyl -

1 ml. Sensorcaine

3 1/2" > 22 Spinal needle.

A-P

oblique

Lat x Depth only.

Inject contrast
c I.V. tubing
Cournay

feel nerve pain
when inject

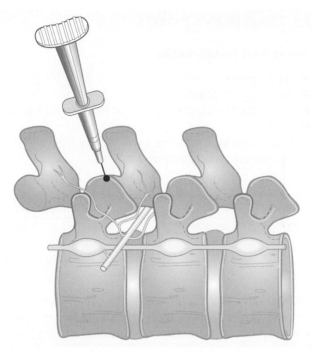

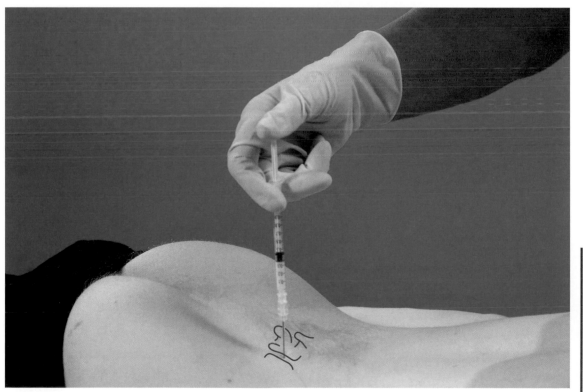

LUMBAR NERVE ROOTS

Nerve root inflammation

Causes and findings
- Spinal stenosis
- Nerve-root entrapment
- Acute or chronic sciatica with or without root signs
- Painful:
  flexion and side bending usually away from painful side
  straight leg raise, slump test

Equipment

Syringe	Needle	Kenalog 40	Lidocaine	Total volume
1 ml	22G 3–3.5 inches (75–90 mm) Spinal	40 mg	Nil	1 ml

Anatomy The lumbar nerve roots emerge obliquely from the vertebral canals between the transverse processes at the level of the spinous process. Draw a vertical line along the centre of the spinous processes and horizontal lines at each spinous level. Two fingers' width laterally along the horizontal line marks entry site for the needle.

Technique
- Patient lies prone over small pillow to aid localization of spinous processes
- Identify spinous process at painful level and mark spot along horizontal line
- Insert needle and pass perpendicularly to depth of about 3 inches (7 cm)
- Aspirate to ensure needle point is not intrathecal
- Inject solution as a bolus around nerve root

Aftercare Patient keeps mobile within pain limits and is reassessed up to 2 weeks later. Repeat as necessary.

Comments This injection can be especially effective when the patient is in severe pain and conservative manual therapy techniques are impossible to administer. It can also be given when caudal epidural has proved unsuccessful – the caudal is technically an easier procedure but the solution might not reach the affected part of the nerve root. The needle must be repositioned if it encounters bone at a distance of about 2 inches (5 cm) as this means it is touching the lamina or facet joint. Equally, repositioning is necessary if the patient complains of sharp 'electric shock' sensation because the needle will be in the nerve root. If clear fluid is aspirated the needle is intrathecal and the procedure must be abandoned, although it can be attempted a few days later. Two levels can be infiltrated at a time. A large patient may require a larger needle.

   If the first level injected does not relieve the symptoms, a level above or below can be tried. This is well worth trying before considering surgery.

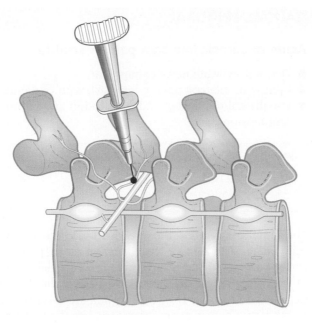

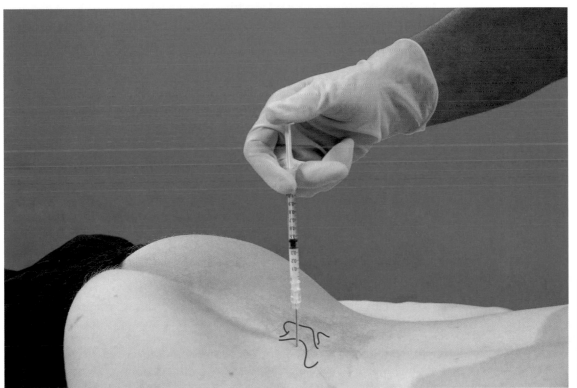

CAUDAL EPIDURAL

Acute or chronic low back pain or sciatica

Causes and findings
- Disc lesion, acute nerve entrapment
- Central or bilateral pain in low back with or without sciatica or root signs
- Usually painful flexion and side flexion away from painful side and nerve root tension signs

Equipment

Syringe	Needle	Kenalog 40	Lidocaine	Total volume
1 ml	21G 1.5 inches (40 mm) Green	40 mg	Nil	1 ml

Anatomy The spinal cord ends at the level of L1 and the thecal sac ends at S2 in most individuals. The aim of this injection is to pass a disinflaming solution through the sacral hiatus and up the canal so that it bathes the posterior aspect of the intervertebral disc, anterior aspect of the dura mater and any affected nerve roots centrally. The sacral cornua are two prominences that can be palpated at the apex of an equilateral triangle drawn from the posterior superior spines on the ileum to the coccyx. There is a thick ligament at the entrance to the canal. The angle of the curve of the canal varies widely and the placement of the needle reflects this.

Technique
- Patient lies prone over small pillow
- Identify sacral cornua at base of imaginary triangle with thumb
- Insert needle between cornua and pass horizontally through ligament
- Pass needle slightly up canal adjusting angle to curve of sacrum
- Aspirate to ensure needle has not penetrated thecal sac or blood vessel
- Slowly inject solution into epidural space
- Keep hand on sacrum to palpate for swelling caused by suprasacral injection

Aftercare The patient lies prone for 10 min and then supine for a further 10 min. He or she can continue to do whatever is comfortable and is reassessed about 10 days later. If the injection has helped it can be repeated at 1- or 2-week intervals as long as improvement continues. The causes of the back pain should then be addressed – weight, posture, work positions, lifting techniques, exercise, abdominal control, etc.

Comments Occasionally the canal is difficult to enter. This might be because of a bifid or very small canal or because the angle of the sacrum is very concave. Reangulation of the needle might be necessary.

If clear fluid or blood is aspirated at any point the procedure is abandoned and attempted a few days later. If the patient feels faint or dizzy during the injection, stop injecting and wait for the symptoms to go. If they do not, abandon the procedure.

Caudal epidural is safe provided[137]:

- there is no allergy to local anaesthetic (not used in this method)
- there is no local sepsis
- the patient is not on anticoagulant therapy

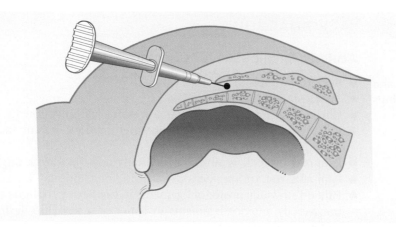

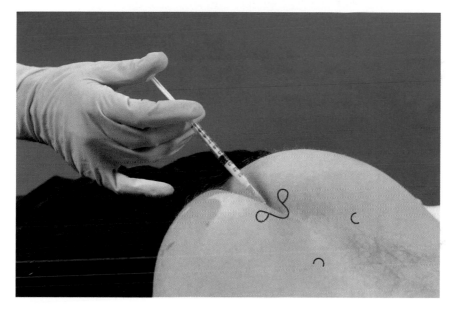

Alternative   If the affected level is higher than the common L5/S1 level, more volume may
approach   be required to reach these levels. In this case we recommend addition of up
to 10 ml of normal saline, depending on the level of the lesion and the size
of the patient[139].

SACROILIAC JOINT

Acute or chronic strain or capsulitis

Causes and findings
- Acute sacroiliitis
- Ankylosing spondylitis
- Chronic ligamentous pain after successful manipulation
- Usually female – often pre- or post-partum or traumatic incident such as fall onto buttocks
- Pain over buttock, groin or occasionally down posterior thigh to calf
- Pain after rest, or long periods of sitting or standing
- Pain on stressing: posterior ligaments in hip flexion, oblique adduction and transversely anterior ligaments in Faber or 4 test (hip flexion, abduction and external rotation)

Equipment

Syringe	Needle	Kenalog 40	Lidocaine	Total volume
2 ml	22G 3–3.5 inches (75–90 mm) Spinal	20 mg	1.5 ml 2%	2 ml

Anatomy
The sacroiliac joint surfaces are angled obliquely posteroanteriorly, with the angle being more acute in the female. The dimples at the top of the buttocks indicate the position of the posterior superior iliac spines. The easiest entry point is usually found in a dip just below and slightly medial to the spines.

Technique
- Patient lies prone over small pillow
- Identify and mark posterior superior iliac spine on affected side
- Insert needle a thumb's width medial and just below this bony landmark at level of second sacral spinous process
- Angle needle obliquely antero-laterally at an angle of about 45°
- Pass needle between sacrum and ilium until a ligamentous resistance is felt.
- Inject solution as a bolus within joint if possible, or pepper posterior capsule

Aftercare
Movement within the pain-free range is encouraged – a lunging motion with the foot up on a chair can help relieve pain, as can moderate walking. The patient should avoid hip abduction positions and sit correctly. A temporary belt is worn if the joint is unstable, and sclerosing injections can be given to increase stability.

Comments
This is not a very common injection; usually manipulation, mobilization and exercise techniques clear the majority of chronic sacroiliac joint symptoms.

The needle often comes up against bone when attempting this injection and then has to be manoeuvred around to allow for the variations in bony shape before entering the joint space.

It is unusual to have to repeat this injection and the joint can often be successfully manipulated if necessary a week later if necessary.

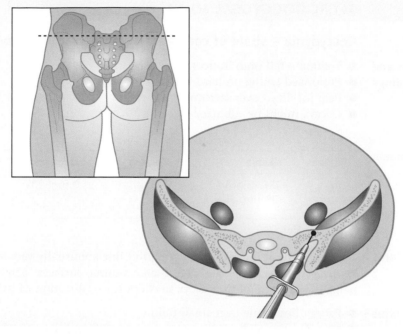

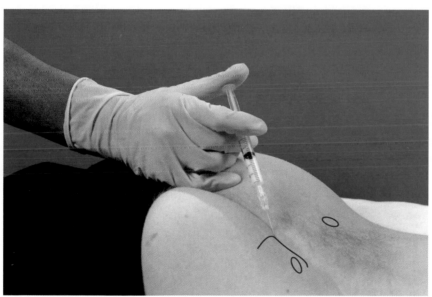

SACROCOCCYGEAL JOINT

Coccydynia – strain of coccygeal ligaments, subluxation

Causes and findings
- Trauma – fall onto buttock
- Prolonged sitting on hard surfaces
- Pain localized over sacrococcygeal joint
- Coccyx might be subluxed

Equipment

Syringe	Needle	Kenalog 40	Lidocaine	Total volume
1 ml	23G 1 inch (25 mm) Blue	20 mg	0.5 ml 2%	1 ml

Anatomy   The ligaments at the sacrococcygeal joint line are usually very tender and can be palpated both on the dorsal and ventral surfaces. The gloved finger palpates the angle of the coccyx to check for subluxation of the bone.

Technique
- Patient lies prone over small pillow
- Identify and mark tender site on dorsum of coccyx at joint line
- Insert needle down to touch bone
- Pepper solution around into tender ligaments

Aftercare   Advise patient to avoid sitting on hard surfaces and to use a ring cushion. At follow-up 2 weeks later, manipulation of the coccyx might be necessary to correct any subluxation; the anti-inflammatory effect of the steroid enables this to be performed with less discomfort. The gloved finger is inserted into the rectum and a firm anteroposterior movement applied. Sometimes an audible click can be heard and some days later the relief of pain is apparent.

Comments   Pain in this area can be symptomatic of psychological or psychosexual distress, in which case the appropriate treatment/advice is required. With somatic pain the protocol above appears to work either well or not at all. Surgery is not usually indicated or particularly successful.

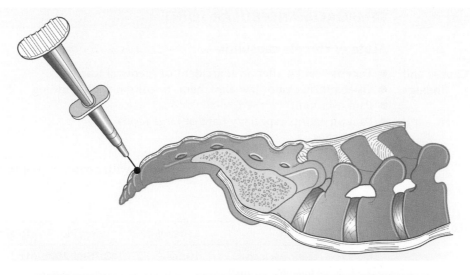

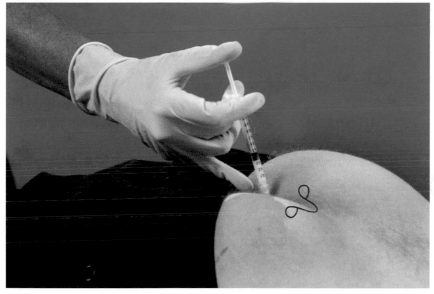

TEMPOROMANDIBULAR JOINT

Acute or chronic capsulitis

Causes and findings
- Trauma – often after a car accident or meniscal tear
- Osteoarthritis, poor jaw alignment, nocturnal teeth grinding
- Pain over joint
- Pain on eating, especially hard or large foods
- Headaches
- Painful:
  - opening, deviation or protrusion of jaw with asymmetry of movement
  - clicking or locking

Equipment

Syringe	Needle	Kenalog 40	Lidocaine	Total volume
1 ml	25G 0.5 inch (16mm) Orange	10mg	0.75 ml 2%	1 ml

Anatomy The temporomandibular joint space can be palpated just in front of the ear as the patient opens and closes the mouth. A meniscus lies within the joint and the needle must be placed below this to enter the joint space. The joint can be infiltrated most easily when the jaw is held wide open.

Technique
- Patient lies on unaffected side with head supported and mouth held open
- Identify and mark joint space
- Insert needle vertically into inferior compartment of joint space below meniscus
- Inject solution as a bolus

Aftercare The patient should avoid excessive movement of the jaw such as biting on a large apple or hard food. Gentle active movements and isometric exercises are carried out. A guard to prevent grinding the teeth at night and/or the advice of an orthodontist might be helpful.

Comments It might be necessary to manoeuvre the needle about to avoid the meniscus.

If the meniscus is displaced, reduction by manipulation should be attempted about 1 week after giving the injection when the inflammation has subsided.

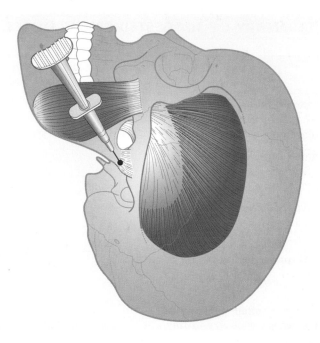

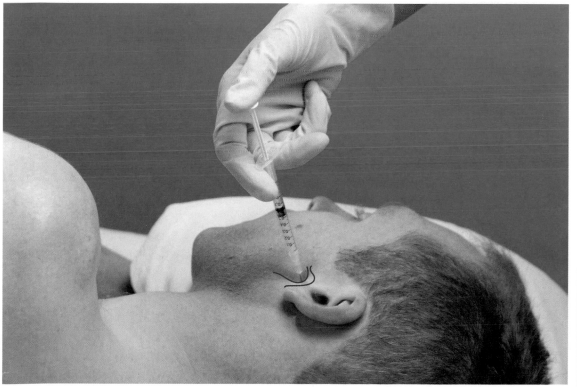

SUMMARY OF SUGGESTED SPINAL DOSES

Syringe	Needle	Kenalog 40	Lidocaine	Total volume
Cervical facet joints: acute or chronic capsulitis				
1 ml	21G 1.5–2 inches (40–50 mm) Green	20 mg		0.5 ml
Lumbar facet joints: chronic capsulitis				
1 ml	22G 3–3.5 inches (75–90 mm) Spinal	40 mg		1 ml
Lumbar nerve roots: nerve root inflammation				
1 ml	22G 3–3.5 inches (75–90 mm) Spinal	40 mg		1 ml
Caudal epidural: acute or chronic low back pain or sciatica				
1 ml	21G 1.5 inches (40 mm) Green	40 mg		1 ml
Sacroiliac joint: acute or chronic strain or capsulitis				
2 ml	22G 3–3.5 inches (75–90 mm) Spinal	20 mg	1.5 ml 2%	2 ml
Sacrococcygeal joint: coccydynia – strain of coccygeal ligaments, subluxation				
1 ml	23G 1 inch (25 mm) Blue	20 mg	0.5 ml 2%	1 ml
Temporomandibular joint: acute or chronic capsulitis				
1 ml	25G 0.5 inch (16 mm) Orange	10 mg	0.75 ml 2%	1 ml

Appendix 1 INJECTION SURVEY

PERIPHERAL JOINT AND SOFT TISSUE INJECTIONS GIVEN IN GENERAL PRACTICE 1991–2004

DR STEPHEN LONGWORTH MBChB MSc FRCGP DM-S Med DPCR FSOM

	Number of injections	%	
Shoulder	1538	39	Upper limb 70%
Elbow	464	12	
Wrist/hand	736	19	
Hip	237	6	Lower limb 30%
Knee	696	18	
Ankle/foot	226	6	
Grand total	3897	100	

TOP SIX INJECTIONS

Injection	Number performed	As percentage of total peripheral injections
Chronic subdeltoid bursitis	801	20%
Shoulder capsulitis	485	
Knee osteoarthritis	464	
Tennis elbow	336	
Trigger digits	209	
Carpal tunnel syndrome	204	
Total	2499	65%

Appendix 2 WEBSITES

The International League of Associations for Rheumatology (ILAR) 'Gateway to world rheumatology' (www.ilar.org) is an excellent place to start, with comprehensive links to other sites and on-line journals. Other sites/addresses of interest are:

American Journal of Sports Medicine:	www.journal.ajsm.org
Annals of the Rheumatic Diseases:	www.ard.bmjjournals.com
Arthritis and Rheumatism:	www.interscience.wiley.com/cgi-bin/jhome/76509746
Bandolier:	www.jr2.ox.ac.uk/bandolier
Best Practice and Research Clinical Rheumatology:	www.clinexprheumatol.org
British Institute of Musculoskeletal Medicine:	www.bimm.org.uk
British Journal of Sports Medicine:	www.bjsm.bmjjournals.com
British Medical Journal:	www.bmj.com
British National Formulary:	www.bnf.org
British Society for Rheumatology:	www.rheumatology.org.uk
Centre For Evidence Based Medicine:	www.cebm.jr2.ox.ac.uk
Clinical Evidence:	www.clinicalevidence.com
Cochrane Library:	www.cochranelibrary.com
Free Books for Doctors:	www.freebooks4doctors.com
Journal of Bone and Joint Surgery (American):	www.ejbjs.org
Journal of Bone and Joint Surgery (British):	www.jbjs.org.uk
Journal of Clinical Rheumatology:	www.jclinrheum.com
Journal of Rheumatology:	www.jrheum.com
Medline National Electronic Library for Health:	www.nelh-pc.nhs.uk
Musculoskeletal Disease Online:	www.jointandbone.org
National Electronic Library for Health:	www.nelh.nhs.uk
National Sports Medicine Institute of the UK:	www.nsmi.org.uk
Oxford Internet Pain Site:	www.jr2.ox.ac.uk/Bandolier/painres/painpag/index.html
Primary Care Rheumatology Society:	www.pcrsociety.com
Resuscitation Council (UK):	www.resus.org.uk
Rheumatology:	www.rheumatology.oupjournals.org
Royal College of Anaesthetists:	www.rcoa.ac.uk
Spine:	www.spinejournal.com
The World of Orthopaedics & Sports Medicine (WorldOrtho):	www.worldortho.com

Access to many of these sites is free for NHS employees, who can obtain an Athens password from their local postgraduate library.

The Association of Chartered Physiotherapists in Orthopaedic Medicine (ACPOM) is a clinical interest group recognized by the Chartered Society of Physiotherapy. Clinicians interested in joining or obtaining more information on injection therapy should visit: acpom.org.uk

TRAINING IN INJECTION THERAPY

Orthopaedic Medicine Seminars conducts courses leading to the Diploma in Injection Therapy for both doctors and physiotherapists. For further information please contact:
Stephanie Saunders, 20 Ailsa Road, Twickenham TW1 1QW
E-mail: stephanie.saunders@virgin.net
www.stephaniesaunders.co.uk

References

1. Anon. Articular and periarticular corticosteroid injection. *Drugs and Therapeutics Bulletin* 1995;33(9):67–70

2. Assendelft WJJ, Hay EM, Adshead R, Bouter LM. Corticosteroid injections for lateral epicondylitis: a systemic overview. *British Journal of General Practice* 1996;46:209–216

3. Van der Hijden GJMG, Van der Windt DAWM, Kleijnen J et al. Steroid injections for shoulder disorders: a systematic review of randomized clinical trials. *British Journal of General Practice* 1996;46:309–316

4. van der Windt DAWM, Koes BW, Deville W et al. Effectiveness of corticosteroid injections versus physiotherapy for treatment of painful stiff shoulder in primary care: randomised trial. *British Medical Journal* 1998;317:1292–1296

5. Dando P, Green S, Price J. *Problems in General Practice – Minor Surgery.* London; The Medical Defence Union 1997

6. Winters JC, Sobel JS, Groenier KH et al. Comparison of physiotherapy manipulation and corticosteroid injection for treating shoulder complaints in general practice: randomised single blind study. *British Medical Journal* 1997;314:1320–1325

7. Hay EM, Paterson SM, Lewis M et al. Pragmatic randomised controlled trial of local corticosteroid injection and naproxen for treatment of lateral epicondylitis of elbow in primary care. *British Medical Journal* 1999;319:964–968

8. Verhaar JAN, Walenkamp GHIM, van Mameren H et al. Local corticosteroid injection versus Cyriax type physiotherapy for tennis elbow. *Journal of Bone and Joint Surgery (Br)* 1995;77:128–132

9. Haslock I, Macfarlane D, Speed C. Intraarticular and soft tissue injections: a survey of current practice. *British Journal of Rheumatology* 1995;34:449–452

10. Marx RG, Bombardier C, Wright JG. What do we know about the reliability and validity of physical examination tests used to examine the upper extremity? *Journal of Hand Surgery* 1999;24A:185–193

11. Bamji AN, Erhardt CC, Price TR, Williams PL. The painful shoulder: can consultants agree? *British Journal of Rheumatology* 1996;35:1172–1174

12. Jones A, Regan M, Ledingham J et al. Importance of placement of intra-articular steroid injections. *British Medical Journal* 1995;307:1329–1330

13. Eustace JA, Brophy DP, Gibney RP et al. Comparison of the accuracy of steroid placement with clinical outcome in patients with shoulder symptoms. *Annals of the Rheumatic Diseases* 1997;56:59–63

14. Hollingworth GR, Ellis RM, Hattersley TS. Comparison of injection techniques for shoulder pain: results of a double blind randomised study. *British Medical Journal* 1983;287:1339–1341

15. Bliddal H. Placement of intra-articular injections verified by mini air-arthrography. *Annals of the Rheumatic Diseases* 1999;58:641–643

16. Kane D, Greaney T, Bresnihan B et al. Ultrasound guided injection of recalcitrant plantar fasciitis. *Annals of the Rheumatic Diseases* 1998;57: 383–384

17. Winters JC, Jorritsma W, Groenier KH et al. Treatment of shoulder complaints in general practice: long term results of a randomised, single blind study comparing physiotherapy, manipulation, and corticosteroid injection. *British Medical Journal* 1999;318:1395–1396

18. Winters JC, Sobel JS, Groenier KH et al. The long term course of shoulder complaints: a prospective study in general practice. *Rheumatology* 1999;38:160–163

19. Bjorkenheim JM, Paavolainen P, Ahovuo J, Slatis P. Surgical repair of the rotator cuff and surrounding tissues. Factors influencing the results. *Clinical Orthopathology* 1988;236:148–153

20. Watson M. Major ruptures of the rotator cuff. The results of surgical repair in 89 patients. *Journal of Bone and Joint Surgery (Br)* 1985;67(4): 618–624

21. ACPOM. *A Clinical Guideline for the Use of Injection Therapy by Physiotherapists*. London; The Chartered Society of Physiotherapy 1999

22. Weale A, Bannister GC. Who should see orthopaedic outpatients – physiotherapists or surgeons? *Annals of the Royal College of Surgeons of England* 1994;77(suppl):71–73

23. Dyce C, Biddle P, Hall K et al. Evaluation of extended role of physio and occupational therapists in rheumatology practice. *British Journal of Rheumatology* 1996 (April, suppl 1: abstracts):130

24. Hattam P, Smeatham. An Evaluation of an orthopaedic screening service in primary care. *British Journal of Clinical Governance* 1999;4(2):45–49

25. Daker-White G, Carr AJ, Harvey I et al. A randomised controlled trial – shifting boundaries of doctors and physiotherapists in orthopaedic outpatient departments. *Journal of Epidemiology and Community Health* 1999;53:643–650

26. Haynes JC Jr. Adrenocorticotrophic hormone; adrenocortical steroids and their synthetic analogues, inhibitors of the synthesis and actions of adrenocortical hormones. In: Goodman AG et al (eds) *Goodman and Gilman's Pharmacological Basis of Therapeutics*, 8th Edn. New York City; Pergamon Press 1990: pp 1431–1469

27. Coombes GM, Bax DE. The use and abuse of steroids in rheumatology. *Reports on the Rheumatic Diseases (Series 3). Practical Problems (No. 8)* 1996

28. Clarke A, Allard L, Braybrooks B. *Rehabilitation in Rheumatology – The Team Approach*. London; Martin Dunitz 1987: pp 147–153

29. Hollander JL, Brown EM, Jester RA et al. Hydrocortisone and cortisone injected into arthritic joints; comparative effects of a use of hydrocortisone as a local anti-arthritis agent. *Journal of the American Medical Association* 1951;147:1269

30. Kendall PH. Triamcinalone hexacetonide – a new corticosteroid for intra-articular therapy. *American Physiology and Medicine* 1967;9:55–58

31. Gray RG, Gottlieb NL. Basic science and pathology: intra-articular corticosteroids, an updated assessment. *Clinical Orthopaedics and Related Research* 1982;177:235–263

32. Creamer P. Intra-articular corticosteroid injections in osteoarthritis: do they work, and if so, how? *Annals of the Rheumatic Diseases* 1997;56: 634–636

33. Goulding NJ. Anti-inflammatory corticosteroids. *Reports on the Rheumatic Diseases (Series 3). Topical Reviews (No. 18)* 1999:1

34. Owen DS. Aspiration and injection of joints and soft tissues. In: Kelly WN et al (eds) *Textbook of Rheumatology*, 5th Edn. New York; WB Saunders 1997: pp 591–608

35. Simone J. The principles of corticosteroid injection therapy in musculoskeletal medicine. *Journal of Orthopaedic Medicine* 1993;15(3):56–58

36. *British National Formulary* No 40 (Sept 2000) p 463 BMA/RPSGB, London

37. Jones A, Doherty M. Intra-articular corticosteroid injections are effective in OA but there are no clinical predictors of response. *Annals of the Rheumatic Diseases* 1996;55:829–832

38. Hochberg MC, Altman RD, Brandt RD et al. Guidelines for the medical management of osteoarthritis. Part II osteoarthritis of the knee. *Arthritis and Rheumatism* 1995;38(11):1541–1546

39. Leadbetter W. Anti-inflammatory therapy in sports injury. *Clinics In Sports Medicine* 1995;14(2):353–410

40. Kirwan JR, Rankin E. Intraarticular therapy in osteoarthritis. *Bailliére's Clinical Rheumatology* 1997;11(4):769–794

41. Dorman T, Ravin T. *Diagnosis and Injection Techniques in Orthopaedic Medicine*. Baltimore, Maryland; Williams and Wilkins 1991: pp 33–34

42. Daley CT, Stanish WD. Soft tissue injuries: overuse syndromes. In: Bull RC (ed) *Handbook of Sports Injuries*. New York; McGraw Hill 1998: p 185

43. Pelletier JP, Pelletier JM. Proteoglycan degrading metalloprotease activity in human osteoarthritis cartilage and the effect of intraarticular steroid injections. *Arthritis and Rheumatism* 1987;30(5):541–549

44. Jubb RW. Anti-rheumatic drugs and articular cartilage. *Reports on the Rheumatic Diseases (Series 2). Topical Reviews (No. 20)* 1992

45. Chard MD, Cawston TE, Riley GP et al. Rotator cuff degeneration and lateral epicondylitis: a comparative histological study. *Annals of the Rheumatic Diseases* 1994;53:30–34

46. Riley GP, Harrall RL, Constant CR et al. Tendon degeneration and chronic shoulder pain: changes in the collagen composition of the human rotator cuff tendons in rotator cuff tendinitis. *Annals of the Rheumatic Diseases* 1994;53:359–366

47. Riley GP, Harrall RL, Constant CR et al. Glycosaminoglycans of human rotator cuff tendons: changes with age and in chronic rotator cuff tendinitis. *Annals of the Rheumatic Diseases* 1994;53:367–376

48. Khan KM, Cook JL, Bonar F et al. Histopathology of common tendinopathies. *Sports Medicine* 1999;27(6):393–408

49. Khan KM, Cook JL, Maffulli N, Kannus P. Where is the pain coming from in tendinopathy? It may be biochemical, not structural in origin. *British Journal of Sports Medicine* 2000;34(2):81–83

50. Blyth T, Hunter JA, Stirling A. Pain relief in the rheumatoid knee after steroid injection: a single blind comparison of hydrocortisone succinate, and triamcinolone acetonide or hexacetonide. *British Journal of Rheumatology* 1994;33(5):461–463

51. Piotrowski M, Szczepanski I, Dmoszynska M. Treatment of rheumatic conditions with local instillation of betamethasone and methylprednisolone: comparison of efficacy and frequency of irritative pain reaction. *Rheumatologia* 1998;36:78–84

52. Birrer RB. Aspiration and corticosteroid injection. *Physiology and Sports Medicine* 1992;20(12):57–71

53. Barry M, Jenner JR. Pain in the neck, shoulder and arm (ABC of Rheumatology). *British Medical Journal* 1995;310:183–186

54. Mens JMA, De Wolf AN, Berkhout BJ, Stam HJ. Disturbance of the menstrual pattern after local injection with triamcinolone acetonide. *Annals of the Rheumatic Diseases* 1998;57:700

55. Drury PL, Howlett TA. Endocrinology. In: Kumar P, Clark M (eds) *Clinical Medicine*, 4th Edn. Edinburgh; W B Saunders 1998: p 941

56. Lazarevic MB, Skosey JL, Djordjevic-Denic G. Reduction of cortisol levels after single intra-articular and intramuscular steroid injection. *American Journal of Medicine* 1995;99(4):370–373

57. Pullar T. Routes of drug administration: intra-articular route. *Prescribers' Journal* 1998;38(2):123–126

58. Taylor HG, Fowler PD, David MJ, Dawes PT. Intra-articular steroids: confounder of clinical trials. *Clinical Rheumatology* 1991;10(1):38–42

59. Fisher M. Treatment of acute anaphylaxis. *British Medical Journal* 1995;311:731–733

60. Ewan PW. Anaphylaxis (ABC of allergies). *British Medical Journal* 1998;316:1442–1445

61. Vervloet D, Durham S. Adverse reactions to drugs (ABC of allergies). *British Medical Journal* 1998;316:1511–1514

62. Wallace WA. (letter) *British Medical Journal* 2000;320 4th March

63. Binder AI, Hazleman BL. Lateral humeral epicondylitis – a study of natural history and the effect of conservative therapy. *British Journal of Rheumatology* 1983;22:73–76

64. Kumar N, Newman R. Complications of intra- and peri-articular steroid injections. *British Journal of General Practice* 1999;49:465–466

65. Newman RJ. Local skin depigmentation due to corticosteroid injections. *British Medical Journal* 1984;288:1725–1726

66. Price R, Sinclair H, Heinrich I, Gibson T. Local injection treatment of tennis elbow – hydrocortisone, triamcinolone and lignocaine compared. *British Journal of Rheumatology* 1991;30:39–44

67. Lanyon P, Regan M, Jones A, Doherty M. Inadvertent intra-articular injection of the wrong substance. *British Journal of Rheumatology* 1997;36: 812–813

68. Gray RG, Tenenbaum J, Gottlieb NL. Local corticosteroid injection therapy in rheumatic disorders. *Seminars in Arthritis and Rheumatism* 1981;10:231–254

69. Cameron G. Steroid arthropathy: myth or reality? *Journal of Orthopaedic Medicine* 1995;17(2):51–55

70. Gosal HS, Jackson AM, Bickerstaff DR. Intra-articular steroids after arthroscopy for osteoarthritis of the knee. *Journal of Bone and Joint Surgery (Br)* 1999;81:952–954

71. Currey HLF, Hull S. Management and referral. In: *Rheumatology for General Practitioners*. Oxford: 1987: p 223

72. Doherty M, Hazleman B, Hutton CW et al. Principles of joint aspiration and steroid injection. In: *Rheumatology Examination and Injection Techniques*. London; WB Saunders 1992: pp 123–127

73. Cooper C, Kirwan JR. Risks of corticosteroid therapy. *Clinical Rheumatology* 1990;19:305–332

74. Smith AG, Kosygan K, Williams H, Newman RJ. Common extensor tendon rupture following corticosteroid injection for lateral tendinosis of the elbow. *British Journal of Sports Medicine* 1999;33:423–425

75. Shrier I, Gordon O. Achilles tendon: are corticosteroid injections useful or harmful? *Clinical Journal of Sports Medicine* 1996;6:245–250

76. Mahler F, Fritsch YD. Partial and complete ruptures of the Achilles tendon and local corticosteroid injections. *British Journal of Sports Medicine* 1992;26:7–14

77. Acevedo JI, Beskin JL. Complications of plantar fascia rupture associated with corticosteroid injection. *Foot and Ankle International* 1998;19:91–97

78. Fredberg U. Local corticosteroid injection in sport: review of literature and guidelines for treatment. *Scandinavian Journal of Medicine and Science in Sport* 1997;7:131–139

79. Cyriax JH, Cyriax PJ. Principles of treatment. In: *Illustrated Manual of Orthopaedic Medicine*. Butterworths 1983: p 22

80. Read MTF. Safe relief of rest pain that eases with activity in achillodynia by intrabursal or peritendinous steroid injection: the rupture rate was not increased by these steroid injections. *British Journal of Sports Medicine* 1999;33:134–135

81. Mottram DR (ed). *Drugs in Sport*, 2nd Edn. London: E & FN Spon 1996

82. Hughes RA. Septic arthritis. *Reports on the Rheumatic Diseases (Series 3). Practical Problems (No. 7)* 1996:1

83. Hollander JL. Intrasynovial corticosteroid therapy in arthritis. *Maryland State Medical Journal* 1970;19:62–70

84. Seror P, Pluvinage P, Lecoq F et al. Frequency of sepsis after local corticosteroid injection (an inquiry on 1,160,000 injections in rheumatological private practice in France). *Rheumatology* 1999;38:1272–1274

85. von Essen R, Savolainen HA. Bacterial infection following intra-articular injection. *Scandinavian Journal of Rheumatology* 1989;18:7–12

86. Case History 1: Inadequate asepsis? *Journal of the Medical Defence Union* 1995;11(1):11

87. Gardner GC, Weisman MH. Pyarthrosis in patient with rheumatoid arthritis; a report of 13 cases and a review of the literature from the past 40 years. *American Journal of Medicine* 1990;88:503–511

88. Knight DJ, Gilbert FJ, Hutchison JD. Lesson of the week: septic arthritis in osteoarthritic hips. *British Medical Journal* 1996;313:40–41

89. Ryan MJ, Kavanagh R, Wall PG, Hazleman BL. Bacterial joint infections in England and Wales: analysis of bacterial isolates over a four year period. *British Journal of Rheumatology* 1997;36:370–373

90. Tramer MR, Moore RA, Reynolds JM, McQuay HJ. Quantitative estimation of rare adverse events which follow a biological progression: a new model applied to chronic NSAID use. *Pain* 2000;85:169–182

91. *British National Formulary* No 40 (Sept 2000) p 582 BMA/RPSGB, London

92. Corrigan B, Maitland GD. Management. *Practical Orthopaedic Medicine.* Oxford; Butterworth Heinemann 1983: p 21

93. Kannus P, Jarvinen M, Niittymaki S. Long- or short-acting anesthetic with corticosteroid in local injections of overuse injuries? A prospective, randomized, double-blind study. *International Journal of Sports Medicine* 1990;11(5):397–400

94. Soluaborn S et al. Cortisone injection with anaesthetic additives for radial epicondylalgia. *Clinical Orthopaedics & Related Research* 1995;316:99–105

95. Jacobs LGH, Barton MAJ, Wallace WA et al. Intraarticular distension and steroids in the management of capsulitis of the shoulder. *British Medical Journal* 1991;302:1498–1501

96. Mulcahy KA, Baxter AD, Oni OOA, Finlay D. The value of shoulder distension arthrography with intra-articular injection of steroid and local anaesthetic: a follow-up study. *British Journal of Radiology* 1993;67:263–266

97. *British National Formulary* No 50. (Sept 2005) pp 503, 504, 511, 640 BMA/RPSGB, London

98. Watts RW, Silagy CA. A meta-analysis on the efficacy of epidural corticosteroids in the treatment of sciatica. *Anaesthesia and Intensive Care* 1995;23:564–569

99. McQuay HJ, Moore RA. Epidural steroids for sciatica. *Anaesthesia and Intensive Care* 1996;24:284–285 (letter)

100. Anon. Hyaluronan or hylans for knee osteoarthritis? *Drugs and Therapeutics Bulletin* 1999;37(9):71–72

101. Gado K, Emery P. Intra-articular guanethidine injection for resistant shoulder pain: a preliminary double blind study of a novel approach. *Annals of the Rheumatic Diseases* 1996;55:199–201

102. Heuft-Dorenbosch LLJ, deVet HCW, van der Linden S. Yttrium radiosynoviorthesis in the treatment of knee arthritis in rheumatoid arthritis: a systematic review. *Annals of the Rheumatic Diseases* 2000;59:583–586

103. Aronson JK. Where name and image meet – the argument for 'adrenaline'. *British Medical Journal* 2000;320:506–509

104. Cawley PJ, Morris IM. A study to compare the efficacy of two methods of skin preparation prior to joint injection. *British Journal of Rheumatology* 1992;31:847–848

105. Dacre JE, Beeney N, Scott DL. Injections and physiotherapy for the painful stiff shoulder. *Annals of the Rheumatic Diseases* 1989;48:322–325

106. Smith RW et al. Methods of skin preparation prior to intra-articular injection. (letter) *British Journal of Rheumatology* 1993;32(7):648

107. Handwashing Liaison Group. Hand washing. *British Medical Journal* 1999;318:686

108. Hartley JC, Mackay AD, Scott GM. Wrist watches must be removed before washing hands. (letter) *British Medical Journal* 1999;318:328

109. Golding DN. Local corticosteroid injections. *Reports on the Rheumatic Diseases (Series 2). Practical Problems* (No. 19) 1991:1

110. Liang MH, Sturock RD. Evaluation of musculoskeletal symptoms. In: Klippel JH, Dieppe PA (eds). *Practical Rheumatology.* London; Mosby 1995: p 11

111. Baker L. *ACPOM Journal* January 1999;7:42–48

112. Department of Health. *Immunisation Against Infectious Diseases,* 2nd Edn. London; HMSO 1994: pp 38–41

113. Ewan PW. Treatment of anaphylactic reactions. *Prescribers' Journal* 1997; 37(3):125–132

114. Sander JWAS, O'Donaghue MF. Epilepsy: getting the diagnosis right. *British Medical Journal* 1997;314:158–159

115. Snashall D. Occupational infections (ABC of work related disorders). *British Medical Journal* 1996;313:553

116. UK Departments of Health. *Guidance for Clinical Health Care Workers: Protection Against Infection with Blood-borne Viruses.* London: HMSO 1998 (Online. Available: http://www.open.gov.uk/doh/chcguid1.htm)

117. Easterbrook P, Ippolito G. Prophylaxis after occupational exposure to HIV. *British Medical Journal* 1997;315:557–558

118. Faher H, Rentsch HV, Gerber NJ et al. Knee effusion and reflex inhibition of the knee joint. *Journal of Bone and Joint Surgery (Br)* 1988;70:635–637

119. Spencer J et al. Knee joint effusion and quadriceps reflex inhibition in man. *Archives of Physical and Medical Rehabilitation* 1984;65:171–177

120. Weitoft T, Uddenfeldt P. Importance of synovial fluid aspiration when injecting intra-articular corticosteroids. *Annals of the Rheumatic Diseases* 2000;59:233–235

121. Dieppe P, Swan A. Identification of crystals in synovial fluid. *Annals of the Rheumatic Diseases* 1999;58:261–263

122. Shmerling RH, Delbanco TL, Tosteson AN, Trentham DE. Synovial fluid tests – what should be ordered? *Journal of the American Medical Association* 1990;264:1009–1014

123. Von Essen R, Holtta A. Improved method of isolating bacteria from joint fluids by the use of blood culture bottles. *Annals of the Rheumatic Diseases* 1986;45:454–457

124. Stell IM, Gransden WR. Simple tests for septic bursitis: comparative study. *British Medical Journal* 1998;316:1877

125. Varley GW, Needoff M, Davis TR, Clay NR. Conservative management of wrist ganglia: aspiration versus steroid infiltration. *Journal of Hand Surgery (Br)* 1997;22(5):636–637

126. Jones D, Chattopadhyay. Suprascapular nerve block for the treatment of frozen shoulder in primary care: a randomized trial. *British Journal of General Practice* 1999;49:39–41

127. Samanta A, Beardsley J. Sciatica: which intervention? *British Medical Journal* 1999;319:302–303

128. Bush K, Hillier S. A controlled study of caudal epidural injections of triamcinolone plus procaine for the management of intractable sciatica. *Spine* 1991;16(5):572–575

129. Koes B, Scholten RPM, Mens JMA, Bouter LM. Efficacy of epidural steroid injections for low back pain and sciatica: a systematic review of randomised clinical trials. *Pain* 1995;63:279–288

130. Carette S, Leclaire R, Marcoux S et al. Epidural corticosteroid injections for sciatica due to herniated nucleus pulposus. *New England Journal of Medicine* 1997;336(23):1634–1640

131. Slosar PJ, White AH, Wetzel FT. Controversy – the use of selective nerve root blocks: diagnostic, therapeutic or placebo? *Spine* 1998;20:2253–2256

132. Riew KD, Yin Y, Gilula L et al. The effect of nerve root injections on the need for operative treatment of lumbar radicular pain. A prospective, randomised, controlled, double blind study. *Journal of Bone and Joint Surgery (America)* 2000;82A:1589–1593

133. Nelemans PJ, de Bie RA, de Vet HCW, Sturmans F. Injection therapy for subacute and chronic benign low back pain (Cochrane Review). In: The Cochrane Library, Issue 4, 2000. Oxford: Update Software

134. Carette S, Marcoux S, Truchon R et al. A controlled trial of corticosteroid injections into facet joints for chronic low back pain. *New England Journal of Medicine* 1991;325(14):1002–1007

135. Ferner RE. Prescribing licensed medicines for unlicensed indications. *Prescribers' Journal* 36(2):73–78

136. Wildsmith JA. Routes of drug administration: 6. Intrathecal and epidural injection. *Prescribers' Journal* 36(2):110–115

137. Price CM, Rogers PD, Prosser ASJ, Arden NK. Comparison of the caudal and lumbar approaches to the epidural space. *Annals of the Rheumatic Diseases* 2000:879–882

138. Cyriax J. Epidural injection. In: *Textbook of Orthopaedic Medicine*, Vol 2, 11th Edn. London; Bailliére Tindall 1984: p 178

139. Bryan BM, Lutz C, Lutz GE. Fluoroscopic assessment of epidural contrast spread after caudal injection. *Journal of Orthopaedic Medicine* 2000;22(2):38–41

140. Dorman T, Ravin T. Treatment. In: *Diagnosis and Injection Techniques in Orthopaedic Medicine*. Baltimore, Maryland; Williams and Wilkins 1991: p. 34

141. Dechow E, Davies RK, Carr AJ, Thompson PW. A randomised, double blind, placebo controlled trial of sclerosing injections in patients with chronic low back pain. *Rheumatology* 1999;38:1255–1259

142. Department of Health. *The NHS Plan. A plan for investment. A plan for reform.* London: The Stationery Office; 2000

143. Hugate R, Pennypacker J, Saunders M, Juliano P. The effects of intra-tendinous and retrocalcaneal intrabursal injections of corticosteroid on the biomechanical properties of rabbit Achilles tendons. *Journal of Bone and Joint Surgery (America)* 2004;86:794–801

144. Johnston SL, Unsworth J. Clinical review; Lesson of the week. Adrenaline given outside the context of life threatening allergic reactions. *British Medical Journal* 2003;326:589–590

145. Pumphrey RSH. Lessons for management of anaphylaxis from a study of fatal reactions. *Clinical and Experimental Allergy* 2000;30:1144–1150

146. Project Team of the Resuscitation Council (UK). Emergency medical treatment of anaphylactic reactions. *Journal of Accident and Emergency Medicine* 1999;16:243–247

147. Glattes RC, Spindler KP, Blanchard GM et al. A simple, accurate method to confirm placement of intra-articular knee injection. *American Journal of Sports Medicine* 2004;32:1029

148. Hoving JL, Buchbinder R, Green S et al. How reliably do rheumatologists measure shoulder movement? *Annals of the Rheumatic Diseases* 2002;61(7):612–616

149. Haynes RB, Devereaux PJ, Guyatt GH. Physicians' and patients' choices in evidence based practice. *British Medical Journal* 2002;324:1350

150. Cluff R, Mehio A, Cohen S et al. The technical aspects of epidural steroid injections: a national survey. *Anesthesia and Analgesia* 2002;95:403–408

151. Jackson DW, Rettig A, Wiltse LL. Epidural cortisone injections in the young athletic adult. *American Journal of Sports Medicine* 1980;8(4):239–243

152. Valat J-P, Giraudeau B, Rozenberg S et al. Epidural corticosteroid injections for sciatica: a randomised, double blind, controlled clinical trial. *Annals of the Rheumatic Diseases* 2003;62:639–643

153. Arden NK, Reading I, Thomas L et al. Epidural corticosteroid injections offer no sustained benefit for patients with sciatica: A randomised controlled trial. *Proceedings of the American College of Rheumatologists, 66th Annual Scientific Meeting* 2002; abstract 530

154. Buttermann GR. Treatment of lumbar disc herniation: epidural steroid injection compared with discectomy; a prospective, randomized study. *Journal of Bone and Joint Surgery (America)* 2004;86:670–679

155. Nørregaard J, Krogsgaard MR, Lorenzen T, Jensen EM. Diagnosing patients with longstanding shoulder joint pain. *Annals of the Rheumatic Diseases* 2002;61:646–649

156. Goupille P, Giraubeau B, Conrozier T et al. *Presentation: Safety and efficacy of intra-articular injection of interleukin-1 receptor agonist in patients with painful osteoarthritis of the knee: a multicenter, double-blind study.* Orlando, FL: American College of Rheumatology: 2003 meeting; 23–28 October 2003: Abstract 1822

157. Likar R, Schafer M, Paulak F et al. Intra-articular morphine analgesia in chronic pain patients with osteoarthritis. *Anesthesia and Analgesia* 1997;84:1313–1317

158. Hasso N, Maddison PJ, Breslin A. Intra-articular methotrexate in knee synovitis. *Rheumatology* 2004;43:779–782

159. Swan A, Amer H, Dieppe P. The value of synovial fluid assays in the diagnosis of joint disease: a literature survey. *Annals of the Rheumatic Diseases* 2002;61:493–498

160. Weiker GG, Kuivila TE, Pippinger CE. Serum lidocaine and bupivacaine levels in local technique knee arthroscopy. *American Journal of Sports Medicine* 1991;19(5):499–502

161. Gill SS, Gelbke MK, Matson SL et al. Fluoroscopically guided low-volume peritendinous corticosteroid injection for Achilles tendinopathy; a safety study. *Journal of Bone and Joint Surgery (America)* 2004;86:802–806

162. Weitoft T, Ronnblom L. Randomised controlled study of post-injection immobilisation after intra-articular glucocorticoid treatment for wrist synovitis. *Annals of the Rheumatic Diseases* 2003;62(10):1013–1015

163. Horlocker TT, Bajwa ZH, Ashraf Z et al. Risk assessment of hemorrhagic complications associated with non-steroidal anti-inflammatory medications in ambulatory pain clinic patients undergoing epidural steroid injection. *Anesthesia and Analgesia* 2002;95:1691–1697

164. Arroll B, Goodyear-Smith F. Corticosteroid injections for osteoarthritis of the knee: meta-analysis. *British Medical Journal* 2004;328:869

165. Raynauld J, Buckland-Wright C, Ward R et al. Safety and efficacy of long-term intraarticular steroid injections in osteoarthritis of the knee. *Arthritis and Rheumatism* 2003;48:370–374

166. Saxena A, Fullem B. Plantar fascia ruptures in athletes. *American Journal of Sports Medicine* 2004;32:662–665

167. McWhorter JW, Francis RS, Heckmann RA. Influence of local steroid injections on traumatized tendon properties; a biomechanical and histological study. *American Journal of Sports Medicine* 1991;19(5):435–439

168. Paavola M, Orava S, Leppilahti J et al. Chronic Achilles tendon overuse injury: Complications after surgical treatment. An analysis of 432 consecutive patients. *American Journal of Sports Medicine* 2000;28:77–82

169. Mair SD, Isbell WM, Gill TJ et al. Triceps tendon ruptures in professional football players. *American Journal of Sports Medicine* 2004;32:431–434

170. Fredburg U. Local corticosteroid injection in sport; review of literature and guidelines for treatment. *Scandinavian Journal of Medicine and Science in Sports* 1997;7(3):131–139

171. Ahmed OA, Ahmed AO, Imran D, Ahmed S. Coughing to distraction. *Anesthesia and Analgesia* 2004;98:343–345

172. Wang C, Lin J, Chang C et al. Therapeutic effects of hyaluronic acid on osteoarthritis of the knee; a meta-analysis of randomized controlled trials. *Journal of Bone and Joint Surgery (America)* 2004;86:538–545

173. American College of Rheumatology subcommittee on osteoarthritis guidelines. Recommendations for the medical management of osteoarthritis of the hip and knee. *Arthritis and Rheumatology* 2000;43:1905–1915

174. Jordan M, Arden NK, Doherty M et al. EULAR Recommendations 2003: an evidence based approach to the management of knee osteoarthritis: Report of a task force of the Standing Committee for International Clinical Studies Including Therapeutic Trials (ESCISIT). *Annals of the Rheumatic Diseases* 2003;62:1145–1155

175. *British National Formulary* No 47 (March 2004) p 477 BMA/RPSGB, London

176. Wiggins ME, Fadale PD, Ehrlich MG, Walsh WR. Effects of local injection of corticosteroids on the healing of ligaments; a follow-up report. *Journal of Bone and Joint Surgery (America)* 1995;77(11):1682–1691

177. Bernardeau C, Bucki B, Liotea F. Acute arthritis after intra-articular hyaluronate injection: onset of effusions without crystal. *Annals of the Rheumatic Diseases* 2001;60:518–520

178. Buchbinder R, Green S, Forbes A et al. Arthrographic joint distension with saline and steroid improves function and reduces pain in patients with painful stiff shoulder: results of a randomised, double blind, placebo controlled trial. *Annals of the Rheumatic Diseases* 2004;63:302–309

179. Helliwell PS. Use of an objective measure of articular stiffness to record changes in finger joints after intra-articular injection of corticosteroid. *Annals of the Rheumatic Diseases* 1997;56:71–73

180. Steroid psychosis after an intra-articular injection. *Annals of the Rheumatic Diseases* 2000;59:926 (Letter)

181. *British National Formulary* No 47. (March 2004) p 347, BMA/RPSGB, London

182. *British National Formulary* No 47. (March 2004) p 346, BMA/RPSGB, London

183. Armstrong RD, English J, Gibson T et al. Serum methylprednisolone levels following intra-articular injection of methylprednisolone acetate. *Annals of the Rheumatic Diseases* 1981;40:571–574

184. Gibson T, Burry HC, Poswillo D, Glass J. Effect of intra-articular corticosteroid injections on primate cartilage. *Annals of the Rheumatic Diseases* 1977;36:74–79

185. *British National Formulary* No 47. (March 2004) p 488, BMA/RPSGB, London

186. *British National Formulary* No 47. (March 2004) p 19, BMA/RPSGB, London

187. International Olympic Committee; Anti-Doping Rules Applicable to the Games of the XXVIII Olympiad in Athens in 2004, available via the internet at *www.olympic.org/uk/organisation/commissions/medical*

188. World Anti-Doping Agency. The world anti-doping code – the 2004 prohibited list (international standard); available via the internet at *www.wada-ama.org*

189. The Football Association Doping Control Programme; Regulations (Season 2004/2005); available via the internet at *www.thefa.com/TheFA/SportsMedical-ExerciseScience/HealthProgrammes*

190. Reeback JS, Chakraborty J, English J. Plasma steroid levels after intra-articular injection of prednisolone acetate in patients with rheumatoid arthritis. *Annals of the Rheumatic Diseases* 1980;39:22–24

191. Luukkainen R, Hakala M, Sajanti E et al. Predictive value of synovial fluid analysis in estimating the efficacy of intra-articular corticosteroid injections in patients with rheumatoid arthritis. *Annals of the Rheumatic Diseases* 1992;51:874–876

192. Balch HW, Gibson JM, El-Ghobarey AF et al. Repeated corticosteroid injections into knee joints. *Rheumatology and Rehabilitation* 1977;16(3): 137–140

193. Bird HA, Ring EF, Bacon PA. A thermographic and clinical comparison of three intra-articular steroid preparations in rheumatoid arthritis. *Annals of the Rheumatic Diseases* 1979;38:36–39

194. Perkins P, Jones AC. Masterclass: Gout. *Annals of the Rheumatic Diseases* 1999;58:611–617

195. Anon. Gout in primary care. *Drugs and Therapeutics Bulletin* 2004; 42(5):39

196. Lane SE, Merry P. Intra-articular corticosteroids in septic arthritis: beneficial or barmy? *Annals of the Rheumatic Diseases* 2000;59:240 (Letter)

197. Pitzalis C. Corticosteroids – a case of mistaken identity? *British Journal of Rheumatology* 1998;37:477–483

198. Padeh S, Passwell JH. Intra-articular corticosteroid injection in the management of children with chronic arthritis. *Arthritis and Rheumatism* 1998;41(7):1210–1214

199. Kullenberg B, Runesson R, Tuvhag R et al. Intraarticular corticosteroid injection: pain relief in osteoarthritis of the hip? *Journal of Rheumatology* 2004;31:2265–2268

200. Bessant R, Steuer A, Rigby S, Gumpel M. Osmic acid revisited: factors that predict a favourable response. *Rheumatology* 2003;42:1036–1043

201. Karlsson J, Sjögren LS, Lohmander LS. Comparison of two hyaluronan drugs and placebo in patients with knee osteoarthritis. A controlled, randomized, double-blind, parallel-design multicentre study. *Rheumatology* 2002;41:1240–1248

202. Zulian F, Martini G, Gobber D et al. Comparison of intra-articular triamcinolone hexacetonide and triamcinolone acetonide in oligoarticular juvenile idiopathic arthritis. *Rheumatology* 2003;42:1254–1259

203. Grayson M. Three infected injections from the same organism. *British Journal of Rheumatology* 1998;37:592–593

204. Lawrence JC, Lilly HA, Kidson A, Davies J. The use of alcoholic wipes for the disinfection of injection sites. *Journal of Wound Care* 1994;3:11–14

205. *British National Formulary* No 47. (March 2004) p 615, BMA/RPSGB, London

206. Cutolo M. The roles of steroid hormones in arthritis. *British Journal of Rheumatology* 1998;37:597–601

207. Smith GR, Jawed S. Effect of music on reducing patient perceived pain whilst undergoing soft tissue and intra-articular injections (Abstract No. 335). *Rheumatology* 2003;42:121–123

208. Huskisson EC, Donnelly S. Hyaluronic acid in the treatment of osteoarthritis of the knee. *Rheumatology* 1999;38:602–607

209. Jawed S, Allard SA. Osteomyelitis of the humerus following steroid injections for tennis elbow. *Rheumatology* 2000;39:923–924 (Letter)

210. Maugars Y, Mathis C, Berthelot JM et al. Assessment of the efficacy of sacroiliac corticosteroid injections in spondylarthropathies: a double-blind study. *British Journal of Rheumatology* 1996;35:767–770

211. Boonen S, Van Distel G, Westhovens R, Dequeker J. Steroid myopathy induced by epidural triamcinolone injection. *British Journal of Rheumatology* 1995;34:385–386

212. Ching DW, Petrie JP, Klemp P, Jones JG. Injection therapy of superficial rheumatoid nodules. *British Journal of Rheumatology* 1992;31:775–777

213. Rees JD, Wojtulewski JA. Systemic reaction to viscosupplementation for knee osteoarthritis. *Rheumatology* 2001;40:1425–1426 (Letter)

214. Ostensson A, Geborek P. Septic arthritis as a non-surgical complication in rheumatoid arthritis: relation to disease severity and therapy. *British Journal of Rheumatology* 1991;30:35–38

215. Pal B, Nash EJ, Oppenheim B et al. Routine synovial fluid culture: is it necessary? Lessons from an audit. *British Journal of Rheumatology* 1997; 36:1116–1117

216. Larsson E, Harris HE, Larsson A. Corticosteroid treatment of experimental arthritis retards cartilage destruction as determined by histology and serum COMP. *Rheumatology* 2004;43(4):428–434

217. Gam A, Schydlowsky P, Rossel I et al. Treatment of 'frozen shoulder' with distension and glucorticoid compared with glucorticoid alone: a randomised controlled trial. *Scandinavian Journal of Rheumatology* 1998; 27(6):425–430

218. Gossec L, Dougados M. Intra-articular treatments in osteoarthritis: from the symptomatic to the structure modifying. *Annals of the Rheumatic Diseases* 2004;63:478–482

219. Sohail MR, Smilack JD. *Aspergillus fumigatus* septic arthritis complicating intra-articular corticosteroid injection. *Mayo Clinic Proceedings* 2004;79(4):578–579

220. Kirschke DL et al. Outbreak of joint and soft-tissue infections associated with injections from a multiple-dose medication vial. *Clinical Infectious Diseases* 2003;36:1369–1373

221. Schumacher HR et al. Pilot investigation of hyaluronate injections for first metacarpal-carpal (MC-C) osteoarthritis. *Journal of Clinical Rheumatology* 2004;10(2):59–62

222. Uthman I, Raynauld JP, Haraoui B. Intra-articular therapy in osteoarthritis. *Postgraduate Medical Journal* 2003;79:449–454

223. Hochberg MC, Perlmutter DL, Hudson JI, et al. Preferences in the management of osteoarthritis of the hip and knee: results of a survey of community-based rheumatologists in the United States. *Arthritis Care and Research* 1996;9:170–176

224. Pelletier JP, Martel-Pelletier J. Protective effects of corticosteroids on cartilage lesions and osteophyte formation in the Pond-Nuki dog model of osteoarthritis. *Arthritis and Rheumatism* 1989;32:181–193

225. Pelletier JP, Mineau F, Raynauld JP, et al. Intraarticular injections with methylprednisolone acetate reduce osteoarthritic lesions in parallel with chondrocyte stromelysin synthesis in experimental osteoarthritis. *Arthritis and Rheumatism* 1994;37:414–423

226. Raynauld JP. Clinical trials: impact of intra-articular steroid injections on the progression of knee osteoarthritis. *Osteoarthritis and Cartilage* 1999; 7:348–349

227. Maheu E. Hyaluronan in knee osteoarthritis. A review of the clinical trials with Hyalgan(R). *European Journal of Rheumatology and Inflammation* 1995;15:17–24

228. Creamer P, Hunt M, Dieppe P. Pain mechanisms in osteoarthritis of the knee: effect of intra-articular anesthetic. *Journal of Rheumatology* 1996;23: 1031–1036

229. Reeves KD, Hassanein KM. Long term effects of dextrose prolotherapy for anterior cruciate ligament laxity. *Alternative Therapies in Health and Medicine* 2003;9(3):58

230. Yelland MJ, Glasziou PP, Bogduk N, Schluter PJ, McKernon M. Prolotherapy injections, saline injections, and exercises for chronic low-back pain: a randomized trial. *Spine* 2004;29(1):9–16; discussion 16

231. van Tulder M, Koes B. Low back pain and sciatica (acute and chronic). In: Clinical Evidence Concise No. 11 (June 2004) p 286–291 BMJ Books (also available on the internet at *www.nelh.nhs.uk/clinicalevidence*)

232. Ongley MJ, Klein RG, Dorman TA, Eck BC, Hubert LJ. A new approach to the treatment of chronic low back pain. *Lancet* 1987;2(8551):143–146

233. Rizzo M, Beckenbaugh RD. Treatment of mucous cysts of the fingers: Review of 134 cases with minimum 2-year follow-up evaluation. *The Journal of Hand Surgery (America)* 2003;28(3):519–525

234. Kim D, Yun Y, Wang J. Nerve-root injections for the relief of pain in patients with osteoporotic vertebral fractures. *Journal of Bone and Joint Surgery (Britain)* 2003;85(2):250–254

235. Tallia AF, Cardone DA. Diagnostic and therapeutic injection of the wrist and hand region. *American Family Physician* 2003;67(4):745–751

236. Nyska M, Kish B, Shabat S et al. The treatment of osteoarthritis of the ankle by intra-articular sodium hyaluronate injection. *Journal of Bone and Joint Surgery (Britain)* 2003;85:246

237. Fufulas EL, Tsintzas D, Gabriilidis B. Treatment of hip osteoarthritis with intra-articular injections of hyaluronic acid. *Journal of Bone and Joint Surgery (Britain)* 2003;85:216

238. Orchard JW. Benefits and risks of using local anaesthetic for pain relief to allow early return to play in professional football. *British Journal of Sports Medicine* 2002;36(3):209–214

239. Avci S, Yilmaz C, Sayli U. Comparison of non-surgical treatment measures for de Quervain's disease of pregnancy and lactation. *Journal of Hand Surgery* 2002;27(A):322–325

240. Alvarez DJ, Rockwell PG. Trigger points: Diagnosis and management. *American Family Physician* 2002;65(4):653–661

241. Hills BA, Ethell MT, Hodgson DR. Release of lubricating synovial surfactant by intra-articular steroid. *British Journal of Rheumatology* 1998;37(6):649–652

242. Black DM, Filak AT. Hyperglycemia with non-insulin-dependent diabetes following intra-articular steroid injection. *The Journal of Family Practice* 1989;28(4):462–463

243. Yangco BG, Germain BF, Deresinski SC. Case report: Fatal gas gangrene following intra-articular steroid injection. *American Journal of the Medical Sciences* 1982;283(2):94–98

244. Hay EM, Thomas E, Paterson SM et al. A pragmatic randomised controlled trial of local corticosteroid injection and physiotherapy for the treatment of new episodes of unilateral shoulder pain in primary care. *Annals of the Rheumatic Diseases* 2003;62:394–399

245. van der Windt DAWM, Bouter LM. Physiotherapy or corticosteroid injection for shoulder pain? *Annals of the Rheumatic Diseases* 2003;62:385–387

246. Carette S et al. Intraarticular corticosteroids, supervised physiotherapy, or a combination of the two in the treatment of adhesive capsulitis of the shoulder: A placebo-controlled trial. *Arthritis and Rheumatism* 2003;48:829–838

247. Carette S. Adhesive capsulitis – research advances frozen in time? *Journal of Rheumatology* 2000;27:1329–1331

248. Marshall S. Carpal tunnel syndrome. In: Clinical Evidence Concise No. 11 (June 2004) pp 271–273, BMJ Books, London (also available on the internet at *www.nelh.nhs.uk/clinicalevidence*)

249. Scott D, Smith C, Lohmander S, Chard J. Osteoarthritis. In: Clinical Evidence Concise No. 11 (June 2004) pp 297–299, BMJ Books, London (also available on the internet at *www.nelh.nhs.uk/clinicalevidence*)

250. Crawford F. Plantar heel pain and fasciitis. In: Clinical Evidence Concise No. 11 (June 2004) pp 300–302, BMJ Books, London (also available on the internet at *www.nelh.nhs.uk/clinicalevidence*)

251. Speed C, Hazleman B. Shoulder pain. In: Clinical Evidence Concise No. 11 (June 2004) pp 304–306, BMJ Books, London (also available on the internet at *www.nelh.nhs.uk/clinicalevidence*)

252. Assendelft W, Green S, Buchbinder R et al. Tennis elbow. In: Clinical Evidence Concise No. 11 (June 2004) pp 307–308, BMJ Books, London (also available on the internet at *www.nelh.nhs.uk/clinicalevidence*)

253. Van der Windt DAWM, Koes BW, De Jong BA, Bouter LM. Shoulder disorders in general practice: Incidence, patient characteristics and management. *Annals of the Rheumatic Diseases* 1995;54:959–964

254. Winters JC, de Jongh AC, van der Windt DAWM et al. The Dutch College of General Practitioners (NHG) practice guideline: shoulder complaints (May 1999) (available on the internet at *www.nhg.artsennet.nl/upload/104/guidelines2*)

255. Croft P. Admissible evidence. *Annals of the Rheumatic Diseases* 1998;57:387–389

256. Hall S, Buchbinder R. Do imaging methods that guide needle placement improve outcome? *Annals of the Rheumatic Diseases* 2004;63:1007–1008

257. Ng LC, Sell P. Outcomes of a prospective cohort study on peri-radicular infiltration for radicular pain in patients with lumbar disc herniation and spinal stenosis. *European Spine Journal* 2004;13(4):325–329

258. Fanciullo GJ, Hanscom B, Seville J et al. An observational study of the frequency and pattern of use of epidural steroid injection in 25,479 patients with spinal and radicular pain. *Regional Anesthesia and Pain Medicine* 2001;26(1):5–11

259. Anon. Medical aspects of drug use in the gym. *Drugs and Therapeutics Bulletin* 2004;42(1):1–4

260. Berger RG, Yount WJ. Immediate 'steroid flare' from intra-articular triamcinolone hexacetonide injection: case report and review of the literature. *Arthritis and Rheumatism* 1990;33(8):1284–1286

261. Gordon GV, Schumacher HR. Electron microscopic study of depot corticosteroid crystals with clinical studies after intra-articular injection. *Journal of Rheumatology* 1979;6:7–14

262. Pharmacokinetics and pharmacodynamics of glucocorticoid suspensions after intra-articular administration. *Clinical Pharmacology and Therapeutics* 1986;39(3):313–317

263. Cassidy JT, Bole GG. Cutaneous atrophy secondary to intra-articular corticosteroid administration. *Annals of Internal Medicine* 1966;65(5):1008–1018

264. Orchard J. The use of local anaesthetic injections in professional football. *British Journal of Sports Medicine* 2001;35:212–213

265. Bamji AM, Dieppe PA, Haslock DI, Shipley ME. What do rheumatologists do? A pilot audit study. *British Journal of Rheumatology* 1990;29:295–298

266. Gossec L, Dougados M. Review: Intra-articular treatments in osteoarthritis: from the symptomatic to the structure modifying. *Annals of the Rheumatic Diseases* 2004;63:478–482

267. Kassimos G, Panayi G, van der Windt DAWM. Differences in the management of shoulder pain between primary and secondary care in Europe: time for a consensus and Author's reply. *Annals of the Rheumatic Diseases* 2004;63:111–112

268. Chustecka Z. Intra-articular injections may introduce skin into affected joint. *Rheumawire*; 7th March 2001 (Available via the internet at *www.jointandbone.org*)

269. Fredberg U, Bolvig L, Pfeiffer-Jensen M et al. Ultrasonography as a tool for diagnosis, guidance of local steroid injection and, together with pressure algometry, monitoring of the treatment of athletes with chronic jumper's knee and Achilles tendinitis: a randomized, double-blind, placebo-controlled study. *Scandinavian Journal of Rheumatology* 2004;33(2):94–101

270. Balint PV, Kane D, Hunter J et al. Ultrasound guided versus conventional joint and soft tissue fluid aspiration in rheumatology practice: a pilot study. *Journal of Rheumatology* 2002;29:2209–2213

271. Razal K, Lee CY, Pilling D et al. Ultrasound guidance allows accurate needle placement and aspiration from small joints in patients with early inflammatory arthritis. *Rheumatology* 2003;42:976–979

272. Speed CA. Corticosteroid injections in tendon lesions. *British Medical Journal* 2001;323:382–386

273. Gormley GJ, Corrigan M, Steele WK et al. Joint and soft tissue injections in the community: questionnaire survey of general practitioners' experiences and attitudes. *Annals of the Rheumatic Diseases* 2003;62:61–64

274. Jolly M, Curran JJ. Underuse of intra-articular and periarticular corticosteroid injections by primary care physicians: discomfort with the technique. *Journal of Clinical Rheumatology* 2003;9(3):187–192

275. Gormley GJ, Steele WK, Stevenson M. A randomised study of two training programmes for general practitioners in the techniques of shoulder injection. *Annals of the Rheumatic Diseases* 2003;62:1006–1009

276. Edwards J, Hannah B, Brailsford-Atkinson K et al. Intra-articular and soft tissue injections: assessment of the service provided by nurses. *Annals of the Rheumatic Diseases* 2002;61:656–657 (Letter)

277. Gaffney K, Ledingham J, Perry JD. Intra-articular triamcinolone hexacetonide in knee osteoarthritis: factors influencing the clinical response. *Annals of the Rheumatic Diseases* 1995;54:379–381

278. Neustadt DH. Intra-articular therapy for RA of the knee – effects of post injection rest regime. *Clinical Rheum Pract* 1985;3:65

279. Chatham W. Intra-articular steroid injection; should we rest the joints? *Arthritis Care and Research* 1989;2(2):70–74

280. Chakravarty K, Pharoah PD, Scott DG. A randomized controlled study of post-injection rest following intra-articular steroid therapy for knee synovitis. *Rheumatology* 1994;33:464–468

281. Richards AJ. Post-injection rest following intra-articular steroid therapy for knee synovitis. *Rheumatology* 1994;33:993–994

282. Pascual E. Management of crystal arthritis. *Rheumatology* 1999;38:912–916

283. Kirwan JR, Haskard DO, Higgens CS. The use of sequential analysis to assess patient preference for local skin anaesthesia during knee aspiration. *British Journal of Rheumatology* 1984;23:210–213

284. Rizzo M, Beckenbaugh RD. Treatment of mucous cysts of the fingers: Review of 134 cases with minimum 2-year follow-up evaluation. *Journal of Hand Surgery (America)* 2003;28(3):519–525

285. Weiss JJ. Intra-articular steroids in the treatment of rotator cuff tear: reappraisal by arthrography. *Archives of Physical Medicine and Rehabilitation* 1981;62(11):555–557

286. Simons DG, Travell JG, Simons LS. *Travell & Simons' Myofascial Pain and Dysfunction: The Trigger Point Manual*, 2nd ed. Baltimore: Williams & Wilkins, 1999, pp 94–173

287. Alvarez D, Rockwell PG. Trigger points: Diagnosis and management. *American Family Physician* 2002;65(4):653–661

288. Smidt N, van der Windt DAWM, Assendelft WJJ et al. Corticosteroid injections, physiotherapy, or a wait and see policy for lateral epicondylitis: a randomised controlled trial. *Lancet* 2002;359:657–662

289. Stitz MY, Sommer HM. Accuracy of blind versus fluoroscopically guided caudal epidural injection. *Spine* 1999;24(13):1371

290. Wang JJ, Ho ST, Lee SC et al. Intra-articular triamcinolone acetonide for pain control after arthroscopic knee surgery. *Anesthesia & Analgesia* 1998;87:1113–1116

291. Yelland MJ, Del Mar C, Pirozzo S, Schoene ML. Prolotherapy injections for chronic low back pain: a systematic review. *Spine* 2004;29(19):2126–2133

292. Ohberg L, Alfredson H. Ultrasound guided sclerosis of neovessels in painful chronic Achilles tendinosis: pilot study of a new treatment. *British Journal of Sports Medicine* 2002;36:173–177

293. Mazur DJ. Influence of the law on risk and informed consent. *British Medical Journal* 2003;327:731–734

294. Rosseland LA, Helgesen KG, Breivik H, Stubhaug A. Moderate-to-severe pain after knee arthroscopy is relieved by intra-articular saline: a randomized controlled trial. *Anesthesia & Analgesia* 2004;98:1546–1551

295. Levine WN, Bergfeld JA, Tessendorf W, Moorman CT. Intramuscular corticosteroid injection for hamstring injuries; a 13-year experience in the National Football League. *American Journal of Sports Medicine* 2000;28:297–300

296. Beiner JM, Jokl P, Cholewicki J, Panjabi MM. The effect of anabolic steroids and corticosteroids on healing of muscle contusion injury. *American Journal of Sports Medicine* 1999;27:2–9

297. Hall S, Buchbinder R. Do imaging methods that guide needle placement improve outcome? *Annals of the Rheumatic Diseases* 2004;63:1007–1008

298. Leopold SS, Battista V, Oliverio JA. Safety and efficacy of intraarticular hip injection using anatomic landmarks. *Clinical Orthopaedics and Related Research* 2001;391:192–197

299. Jackson DW, Evans NA, Thomas BM. Accuracy of needle placement into the intra-articular space of the knee. *Journal of Bone and Joint Surgery (America)* 2002;84:1522–1527

300. Taras JS, Raphael JS, Pan WT, Movagharnia F, Sotereanos DG. Corticosteroid injections for trigger digits: is intrasheath injection necessary? *Journal of Hand Surgery (America)* 1998;23:717–722

301. Pollard MA, Cermak MB, Williams DP, Buck WR. Accuracy of injection into the basal joint of the thumb. *Orthopedics* 2003;(suppl):4

302. Zingas C, Failla JM, Van Holsbeeck M. Injection accuracy and clinical relief of de Quervain's tendinitis. *Journal of Hand Surgery (America)* 1998;23:89–96

303. Naredo E, Cabero F, Beneyto P et al. A randomized comparative study of short term response to injection versus sonographic-guided injection of local corticosteroids in patients with painful shoulder. *Journal of Rheumatology* 2004;31:308–314

304. Kane D, Greaney T, Shanahan M et al. The role of ultrasonography in the diagnosis and management of idiopathic plantar fasciitis. *Rheumatology* 2001;9:1002–1008

305. Shanahan EM, Smith MD, Wetherall M et al. Suprascapular nerve block in chronic shoulder pain: are the radiologists better? *Annals of the Rheumatic Diseases* 2004;63:1035–1040

306. Lewis MP, Thomas P, Wilson LF, Mulholland RC. The 'whoosh' test; a clinical test to confirm correct needle placement in caudal epidural injections. *Anaesthesia* 1992;47(1):57–58

307. Filippuccil E, Farinal A, Carotti M et al. Grey scale and power Doppler sonographic changes induced by intra-articular steroid injection treatment. *Annals of the Rheumatic Diseases* 2004;63:740–743

308. Terslev L, Torp-Pedersen S, Qvistgaard E et al. Estimation of inflammation by Doppler ultrasound: quantitative changes after intra-articular treatment in rheumatoid arthritis. *Annals of the Rheumatic Diseases* 2003;62:1049–1053

309. Bliddal H, Torp-Pedersen S. Use of small amounts of ultrasound guided air for injections. *Annals of the Rheumatic Diseases* 2000;59:926 (Letter)

310. Kamel M, Kotob H. High frequency ultrasonographic findings in plantar fasciitis and assessment of local steroid injection. *Journal of Rheumatology* 2000;27:2139–2141

311. Koski JM. Ultrasound guided injections in rheumatology. *Journal of Rheumatology* 2000;27:2131–2138.

312. van der Windt DAWM, Bouter LM. Physiotherapy or corticosteroid injection for shoulder pain? *Annals of the Rheumatic Diseases* 2003;62:385–387

313. Buchbinder R, Green S. Effect of arthrographic shoulder joint distension with saline and corticosteroid for adhesive capsulitis. *British Journal of Sports Medicine* 2004;38:384–385

314. Edwards J. Intra-articular and soft tissue injections by nurses: preparation for expanded practice. *Nursing Standard* 2000;14(33):43–47

315. Samanta A, Samanta J. Is epidural injection of steroids effective for low back pain? *British Medical Journal* 2004;328:1509–1510

316. Scott A, Khan KM, Cook JL, Duronio V. What is 'inflammation'? Are we ready to move beyond Celsus? *British Journal of Sports Medicine* 2004;38:248–249

317. Scott A, Khan KM, Roberts CR et al. What do we mean by 'inflammation'? A contemporary basic science update for sports medicine. *British Journal of Sports Medicine* 2004;38:372–380

INDEX

ELSEVIER CD-ROM LICENCE AGREEMENT

PLEASE READ THE FOLLOWING AGREEMENT CAREFULLY BEFORE USING THIS PRODUCT. THIS PRODUCT IS LICENSED UNDER THE TERMS CONTAINED IN THIS LICENCE AGREEMENT ('Agreement'). BY USING THIS PRODUCT, YOU, AN INDIVIDUAL OR ENTITY INCLUDING EMPLOYEES, AGENTS AND REPRESENTATIVES ('You' or 'Your'), ACKNOWLEDGE THAT YOU HAVE READ THIS AGREEMENT, THAT YOU UNDERSTAND IT, AND THAT YOU AGREE TO BE BOUND BY THE TERMS AND CONDITIONS OF THIS AGREEMENT. ELSEVIER LIMITED ('Elsevier') EXPRESSLY DOES NOT AGREE TO LICENSE THIS PRODUCT TO YOU UNLESS YOU ASSENT TO THIS AGREEMENT. IF YOU DO NOT AGREE WITH ANY OF THE FOLLOWING TERMS, YOU MAY, WITHIN THIRTY (30) DAYS AFTER YOUR RECEIPT OF THIS PRODUCT RETURN THE UNUSED PRODUCT AND ALL ACCOMPANYING DOCUMENTATION TO ELSEVIER FOR A FULL REFUND.

DEFINITIONS As used in this Agreement, these terms shall have the following meanings:

'Proprietary Material' means the valuable and proprietary information content of this Product including without limitation all indexes and graphic materials and software used to access, index, search and retrieve the information content from this Product developed or licensed by Elsevier and/or its affiliates, suppliers and licensors.

'Product' means the copy of the Proprietary Material and any other material delivered on CD-ROM and any other human readable or machine-readable materials enclosed with this Agreement, including without limitation documentation relating to the same.

OWNERSHIP This Product has been supplied by and is proprietary to Elsevier and/or its affiliates, suppliers and licensors. The copyright in the Product belongs to Elsevier and/or its affiliates, suppliers and licensors and is protected by the copyright, trademark, trade secret and other intellectual property laws of the United Kingdom and international treaty provisions, including without limitation the Universal Copyright Convention and the Berne Copyright Convention. You have no ownership rights in this Product. Except as expressly set forth herein, no part of this Product, including without limitation the Proprietary Material, may be modified, copied or distributed in hardcopy or machine-readable form without prior written consent from Elsevier. All rights not expressly granted to You herein are expressly reserved. Any other use of this Product by any person or entity is strictly prohibited and a violation of this Agreement.

SCOPE OF RIGHTS LICENSED (PERMITTED USES) Elsevier is granting to You a limited, non-exclusive, non-transferable licence to use this Product in accordance with the terms of this Agreement. You may use or provide access to this Product on a single computer or terminal physically located at Your premises and in a secure network or move this Product to and use it on another single computer or terminal at the same location for personal use only, but under no circumstances may You use or provide access to any part or parts of this Product on more than one computer or terminal simultaneously.

You shall not (a) copy, download, or otherwise reproduce the Product or any part(s) thereof in any medium, including, without limitation, online transmissions, local area networks, wide area networks, intranets, extranets and the Internet, or in any way, in whole or in part, except for printing out or downloading nonsubstantial portions of the text and images in the Product for Your own personal use; (b) alter, modify, or adapt the Product or any part(s) thereof, including but not limited to decompiling, disassembling, reverse engineering, or creating derivative works, without the prior written approval of Elsevier; (c) sell, license or otherwise distribute to third parties the Product or any part(s) thereof; or (d) alter, remove, obscure or obstruct the display of any copyright, trademark or other proprietary notice on or in the Product or on any printout or download of portions of the Proprietary Materials.

RESTRICTIONS ON TRANSFER This Licence is personal to You, and neither Your rights hereunder nor the tangible embodiments of this Product, including without limitation the Proprietary Material, may be sold, assigned, transferred or sublicensed to any other person, including without limitation by operation of law, without the prior written consent of Elsevier. Any purported sale, assignment, transfer or sublicense without the prior written consent of Elsevier will be void and will automatically terminate the Licence granted hereunder.

TERM This Agreement will remain in effect until terminated pursuant to the terms of this Agreement. You may terminate this Agreement at any time by removing from Your system and destroying the Product and any copies of the Proprietary Material. Unauthorized copying of the Product, including without limitation, the Proprietary Material and documentation, or otherwise failing to comply with the terms and conditions of this Agreement shall result in automatic termination of this licence and will make available to Elsevier legal remedies. Upon termination of this Agreement, the licence granted herein will terminate and You must immediately destroy the Product and all copies of the Product and of the Proprietary Material, together with any and all accompanying documentation. All provisions relating to proprietary rights shall survive termination of this Agreement.

LIMITED WARRANTY AND LIMITATION OF LIABILITY Elsevier warrants that the software embodied in this Product will perform in substantial compliance with the documentation supplied in this Product, unless the performance problems are the result of hardware failure or improper use. If You report a significant defect in performance in writing to Elsevier within ninety (90) calendar days of your having purchased the Product, and Elsevier is not able to correct same within sixty (60) days after its receipt of Your notification, You may return this Product, including all copies and documentation, to Elsevier and Elsevier will refund Your money. In order to apply for a refund on your purchased Product, please contact the return address on the invoice to obtain the refund request form ('Refund Request Form'), and either fax or mail your signed request and your proof of purchase to the address indicated on the Refund Request Form. Incomplete forms will not be processed. Defined terms in the Refund Request Form shall have the same meaning as in this Agreement.

YOU UNDERSTAND THAT, EXCEPT FOR THE LIMITED WARRANTY RECITED ABOVE, ELSEVIER, ITS AFFILIATES, LICENSORS, THIRD PARTY SUPPLIERS AND AGENTS (TOGETHER 'THE SUPPLIERS') MAKE NO REPRESENTATIONS OR WARRANTIES, WITH RESPECT TO THE PRODUCT, INCLUDING, WITHOUT LIMITATION THE PROPRIETARY MATERIAL. ALL OTHER REPRESENTATIONS, WARRANTIES, CONDITIONS OR OTHER TERMS, WHETHER EXPRESS OR IMPLIED BY STATUTE OR COMMON LAW, ARE HEREBY EXCLUDED TO THE FULLEST EXTENT PERMITTED BY LAW.

IN PARTICULAR BUT WITHOUT LIMITATION TO THE FOREGOING NONE OF THE SUPPLIERS MAKE ANY REPRESENTIONS OR WARRANTIES (WHETHER EXPRESS OR IMPLIED) REGARDING THE PERFORMANCE OF YOUR PAD, NETWORK OR COMPUTER SYSTEM WHEN USED IN CONJUNCTION WITH THE PRODUCT, NOR THAT THE PRODUCT WILL MEET YOUR REQUIREMENTS OR THAT ITS OPERATION WILL BE UNINTERRUPTED OR ERROR-FREE.

EXCEPT IN RESPECT OF DEATH OR PERSONAL INJURY CAUSED BY THE SUPPLIERS' NEGLIGENCE AND TO THE FULLEST EXTENT PERMITTED BY LAW, IN NO EVENT (AND REGARDLESS OF WHETHER SUCH DAMAGES ARE FORESEEABLE AND OF WHETHER SUCH LIABILITY IS BASED IN TORT, CONTRACT OR OTHERWISE) WILL ANY OF THE SUPPLIERS BE LIABLE TO YOU FOR ANY DAMAGES (INCLUDING, WITHOUT LIMITATION, ANY LOST PROFITS, LOST SAVINGS OR OTHER SPECIAL, INDIRECT, INCIDENTAL OR CONSEQUENTIAL DAMAGES ARISING OUT OF OR RESULTING FROM: (I) YOUR USE OF, OR INABILITY TO USE, THE PRODUCT; (II) DATA LOSS OR CORRUPTION; AND/OR (III) ERRORS OR OMISSIONS IN THE PROPRIETARY MATERIAL.

IF THE FOREGOING LIMITATION IS HELD TO BE UNENFORCEABLE, OUR MAXIMUM LIABILITY TO YOU IN RESPECT THEREOF SHALL NOT EXCEED THE AMOUNT OF THE LICENCE FEE PAID BY YOU FOR THE PRODUCT. THE REMEDIES AVAILABLE TO YOU AGAINST ELSEVIER AND THE LICENSORS OF MATERIALS INCLUDED IN THE PRODUCT ARE EXCLUSIVE.

If the information provided In the Product contains medical or health sciences information, it is intended for professional use within the medical field. Information about medical treatment or drug dosages is intended strictly for professional use, and because of rapid advances in the medical sciences, independent verification of diagnosis and drug dosages should be made. The provisions of this Agreement shall be severable, and in the event that any provision of this Agreement is found to be legally unenforceable, such unenforceability shall not prevent the enforcement or any other provision of this Agreement.

GOVERNING LAW This Agreement shall be governed by the laws of England and Wales. In any dispute arising out of this Agreement, you and Elsevier each consent to the exclusive personal jurisdiction and venue in the courts of England and Wales.

Minimum System Requirements
Windows 98, 2000, NT, ME or XP operating system
Mac OS 9.2 or later operating system
800 × 600 pixels screen resolution, millions of colours
256MB RAM
CD-ROM drive
QuickTime version 6 or later

Technical Support
Technical support for this product is available between 7.30 a.m. and 7.00 p.m. CST, Monday through Friday.

Before calling, be sure that your computer meets the minimum system requirements to run this software.

Inside the United States and Canada, call 1-800-692-9010.
Inside the United Kingdom, call 0-0800-6929-0100.
Rest of World, call +1-314-872-8370.
You may also fax your questions to +1-314-523-4932,
or contact Technical Support through e-mail: technical.support@elsevier.com.